THE WHOLE TRUTH ABOUT CONTRACEPTION

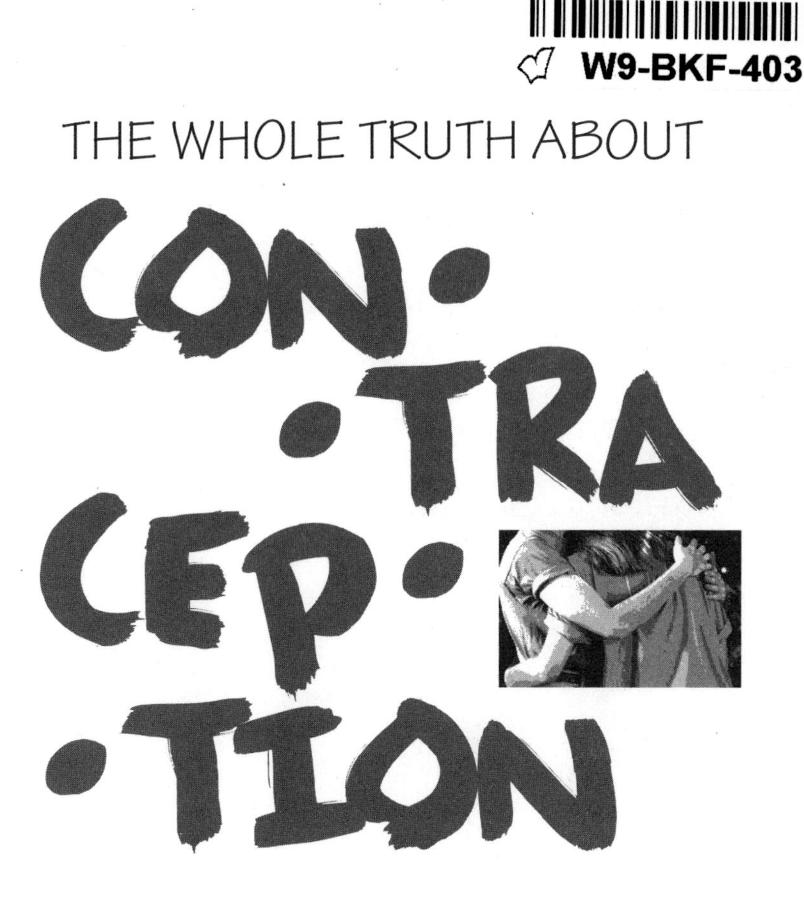

A GUIDE TO SAFE AND EFFECTIVE CHOICES

by Beverly Winikoff, MD, MPH, and Suzanne Wymelenberg

JOSEPH HENRY PRESS
WASHINGTON, D.C. 1997

JOSEPH HENRY PRESS • 2101 Constitution Avenue, N.W. • Washington, D.C. 20418

The Joseph Henry Press, an imprint of the National Academy Press, was created with the goal of making books on science, technology, and health more widely available to professionals and the public. Joseph Henry was one of the founders of the National Academy of Sciences and a leader of early American science.

Library of Congress Cataloging-in-Publication Data

Winikoff, Beverly.
The whole truth about contraception : a guide to safe and effective choices / by Beverly Winikoff, and Suzanne Wymelenberg.
p. cm.
Includes bibliographical references and index.
Summary : A detailed guide to currently available methods of birth control.
ISBN 0-309-05494-X (alk. paper)
1. Contraception—Popular works. [1. Birth control.]
I. Wymelenberg, Suzanne. II. Title.
RG136.2.W54 1997
613.9′4—dc21 97-26488
CIP
AC

Illustrations by Roberto Osti.

Printed in the United States of America.

The ideas, procedures, and suggestions contained in this book are not intended to replace the services of a physician. Many matters regarding your health require medical supervision and you should consult a physician before adopting the procedures described here. Any application of the treatments set forth in this book is at the reader's sole discretion and neither the authors nor the publisher assume any responsibility or liability therefor.

Contents

PART TWO
Hormonal Methods

PART THREE
The Intrauterine Method

PART FOUR
Surgical Methods

PART FIVE
Other Methods of Fertility Control

PART SIX
Other Issues of Birth Control

THE WHOLE TRUTH ABOUT

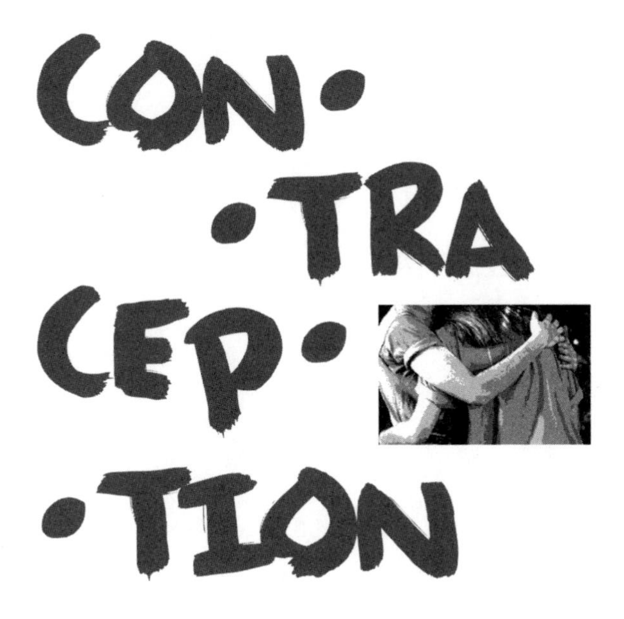

Introduction

Contraception, in one form or another, has been practiced by humans for thousands of years. Before the development of modern methods, women placed ground herbs mixed with oil or honey in their vaginas or inserted sea sponges soaked in lemon juice to act as barriers to conception. For many years douches were used as a popular, although ineffective, method of birth control for women. Since the sixteenth century, men have had the option of using condoms. There is no record of how successful the many methods used in the past actually were, but their prevalence in folklore demonstrates a great interest in controlling fertility by preventing pregnancy.

Men and women want birth control that is safe, effective, affordable, and convenient to use, and today more than ever we have a variety of choices that come close to these ideals. People often need different types of contraceptives to suit the different stages in their lives. A method that is useful for spacing pregnancies, for instance, is not necessarily adequate for the woman who wants to stop childbearing completely. And a contraceptive that works well for someone who has sexual intercourse only occasionally may not be sufficiently effective for those who have sex often.

This book is not written for any one age or lifestyle, but addresses all women and men who are interested in birth control.

Although methods of contraception are very effective, *the surest protection against pregnancy and sexually transmitted diseases is abstinence.*

CONTRACEPTIVE CHOICES IN THE UNITED STATES

Various methods of contraception are available in the United States today, including condoms for men and women; spermicidal foams, gels, and vaginal films; diaphragms and cervical caps; the Pill; IUDs; and fertility awareness methods that rely on periodic abstinence. There are injections that last for 3 months and implants that last 5 years. There is emergency contraception. The most frequently used birth control is female sterilization; the Pill and male condoms are second and third most common.

CONTRACEPTIVES AND SEXUALLY TRANSMITTED DISEASES

Barrier contraceptives, such as condoms and diaphragms, can have an important use beyond birth control—they can also reduce the chance of spreading sexually transmitted diseases (STDs), including AIDS. AIDS is now the leading cause of death for U.S. men between the ages of 25 and 44. It is spread among heterosexuals as well as homosexuals. Today, AIDS is spreading the most rapidly among women, among whom it is a major cause of death. As of early 1997 it was the third leading killer of women of reproductive age, two-thirds of whom were infected through sex.

Anyone who is sexually active can acquire a sexually transmitted disease—even if they have sex only once with an infected person. And anyone who has ever had sex can have an STD without knowing it, no matter how healthy they look or feel. The AIDS virus, HIV, can be present without symptoms for many years after a single sexual encounter with someone who had the virus.

While other STDs seldom kill in this country, they can undermine your health and fertility and be passed on to a baby who is still in the womb. STDs also can lead to pelvic inflammatory disease (PID), which is fairly common today in the United States. PID results when bacteria that is passed from the man to the woman during sex travels to the uterus and the fallopian tubes. (PID also can follow childbirth or abortion.) The infection, inflammation, and scar tissue caused by these microbes can block the delicate fallopian tubes. Blocked or scarred tubes lead to infertility or to tubal (ectopic) pregnancies that can be life threatening. If caught early, most cases of PID can be treated with antibiotics; if neglected or not recognized, the disease can lead to chronic pain, major surgery, or even death.

Unfortunately, most STDs, including AIDS, do not always produce symptoms in their early stages and sometimes not at all. At least 24 different STDs have been identified, including syphilis, gonorrhea, AIDS, genital warts, chlamydia, herpes simplex, and hepatitis B. The germs that cause these diseases can be carried in semen, blood, and other body fluids.

A woman does not need to have sex frequently with an infected person in order to acquire a sexually transmitted disease. Medical researchers have found that a woman has a 50 percent chance of getting gonorrhea from having intercourse *just once* with an infected man. A man has a 25 percent chance of acquiring gonorrhea after a single act of intercourse with an infected woman. Unless a sexually active individual is in a long-term relationship that is mutually faithful, the surest protection against STDs is a barrier contraceptive.

The barrier methods available today are male condoms, female condoms, the diaphragm, and the cervical cap. We know that male condoms plus a spermicide provide excellent protection against bacterial and viral STDs, including AIDS. If used with a spermicide, the diaphragm and cervical cap provide good protection against bacterial diseases, but effectiveness against AIDS, a virus-caused disease, has not been shown. Because the female condom is fairly new, not very much is known about its effectiveness against disease.

The only other protection against these infections is abstinence from sex or a long-term, strictly monogamous relationship between uninfected partners. Unless a person brings a sexually transmitted disease into a relationship, if both partners remain faithful, there is no chance of catching such a disease. When a relationship is on the brink of becoming sexually intimate, some couples have themselves tested for STDs so they do not unknowingly infect their partners.

NOTE: No matter what type of contraceptive you use, it is a good idea to have a Pap smear and a pelvic exam periodically. The Pap test can detect early cancerous cervical changes and the pelvic exam can find other conditions that may not have symptoms.

ABOUT THIS BOOK

The Whole Truth About Contraception is a detailed guide to the methods of birth control currently available in this country, plus a brief review of new methods being developed. Each chapter describes a specific method and provides information to help you choose a contraceptive suited to you and your current situation. Chapters discuss the advantages and disadvantages of each contraceptive, safety concerns, general effectiveness, side effects, costs, and how to obtain and use it.

You will notice that we frequently refer to "practitioners" or "health care providers" instead of physicians in this book. Most family planning services, particularly education and counseling services, are provided by specially trained nonphysicians working in a variety of agencies: health departments, hospitals, Planned Parenthood affiliates, and independent clinics.

As you think about the birth control options available to you, remember that no single method may be ideal or totally reliable. Furthermore, many contraceptives have some side effects and most require a certain amount of care in their use. To choose the right one for you, be thoughtful about the disadvantages as well as the advantages. If you are comfortable with your birth control choice, you are more likely to use it every time and to stick with it. If possible, the decision about what method to choose should be made with your sexual partner. As these chapters demonstrate, it is much easier to use a contraceptive correctly when both of you are involved.

The information in this book is as up-to-date as we have been able to make it. We discuss only birth control methods that are available now or show every promise of being available soon. Many of the methods discussed in the following chapters require a visit to a health care practitioner. You can make such a visit an opportunity to have a checkup of your general health, to get answers to the questions you have, and to obtain the latest information.

If you are under 18, be reassured that clinics and physicians will not automatically inform your parents or a guardian that you have been asking about birth control. To be absolutely certain, do not be afraid to ask directly about the policy on this issue.

A word of caution: Reports appear in the media about this or that newly discovered danger related to a particular contraceptive. Such early reports often are not substantiated by further research, or the danger may apply only to a small, special group of those who use the method. When such reports are publicized, it is important not to panic, but to continue using your method until you and your doctor have had a chance to learn more about the particular study and whether it applies to you. *Unless you want to get pregnant, it is important not to stop using a contraceptive even for a short time, unless you have begun to use another method.*

1

The Biology of Reproduction

To understand the different methods of birth control that are available today and to choose the best one for you, you will need to know something about the male and female reproductive systems and the process of conception. This chapter outlines how the systems work and how conception takes place.

THE MALE

The sexual organs of the male consist of the penis, scrotum, and testicles (on the outside), and the epididymis, the vas deferens, the prostate, and the urethra (on the inside) (see Figures 1.1 and 1.2).

The *penis* is composed mostly of soft, spongy tissue packed with a network of tiny blood vessels. Two sections of this tissue lie side by side along the upper part of the penis and help anchor it to the pubic bones. A third section lies underneath the entire length of the penis. At the tip this particular section broadens and forms the *glans*. The penis is covered with loose skin; in addition, on an uncircumcised penis, a fold of this skin, the foreskin, hangs over the glans. When a man is aroused sexually, the valve system in the blood vessels of the penis closes the usual exits in the blood network. As a

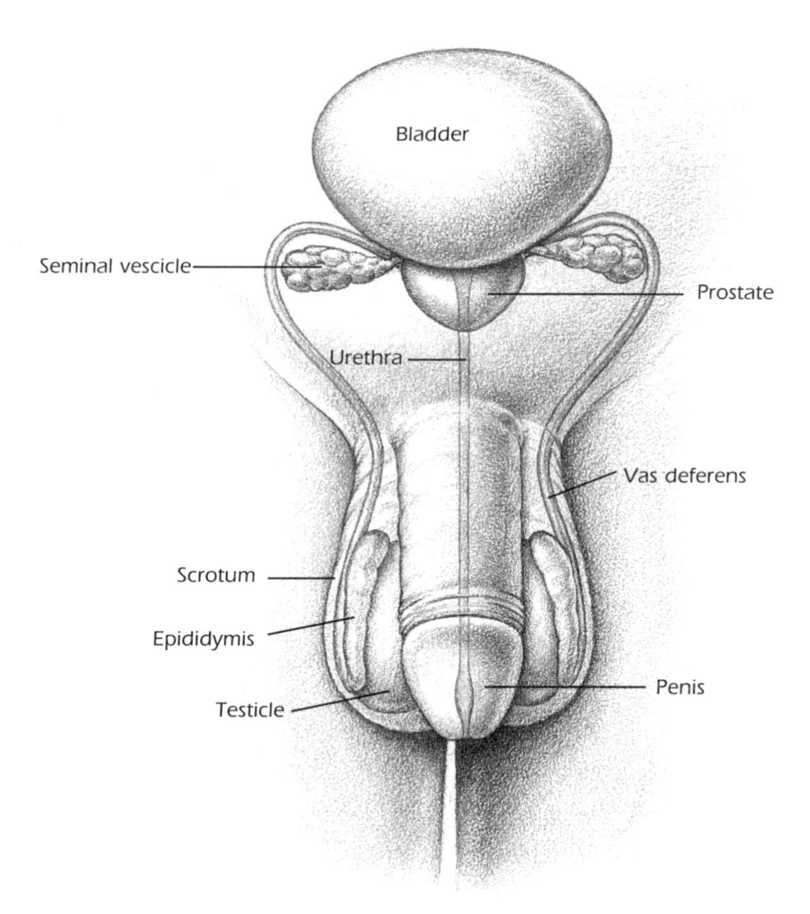

FIGURE 1.1 The Male Reproductive System (Frontal View)

result, the spongy tissues fill with blood and the penis becomes hard and erect, allowing it to penetrate the vagina.

The *scrotum* is the pouch of skin that hangs behind the penis and holds the testicles. It is sensitive to sexual stimulation and to changes in the temperature outside the body. The scrotum's function is to keep the testicles at the right temperature for producing sperm. It sometimes tightens up to hold the testicles snug against the body to keep them warm. At other times it becomes very loose, so the testicles can cool off.

The two *testicles*, or *testes*, are composed of delicate, tiny, tightly

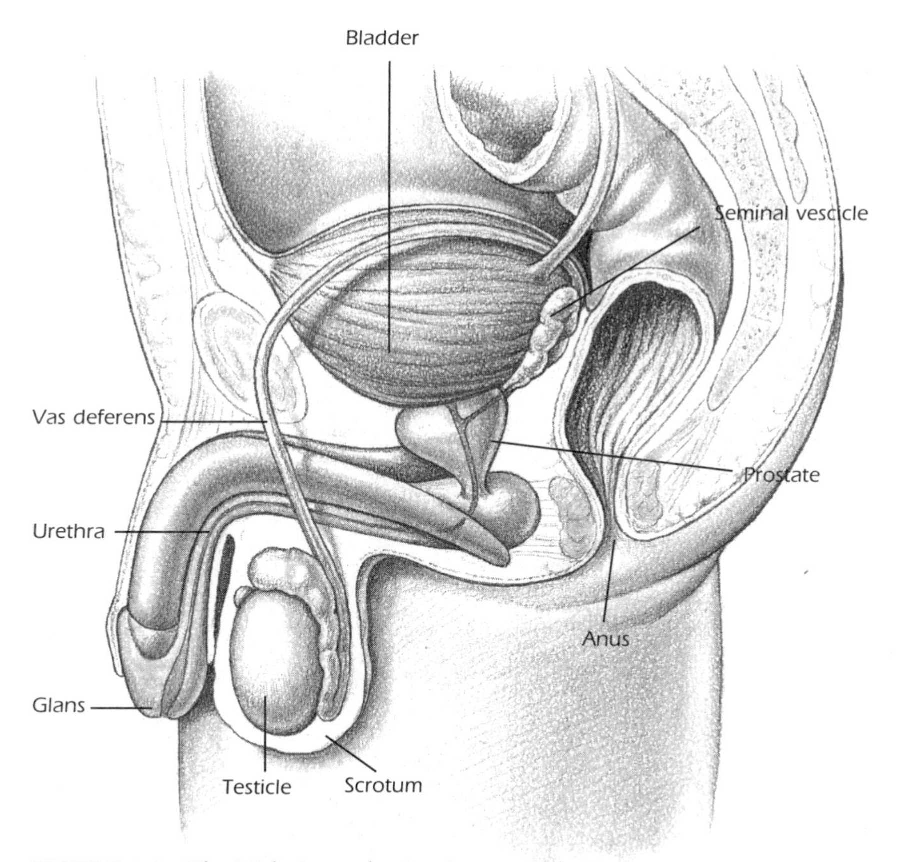

FIGURE 1.2 The Male Reproductive System (Side View)

coiled tubes that are lined with cells designed to manufacture either sperm or hormones. In the fetus, the testicles are formed in the abdomen and by the time of birth have descended into the scrotum. If the testes fail to descend or do not develop completely, this sometimes reduces sperm production and can be a cause of infertility.

During the teen years, the testicles grow and certain cells within the coil of tubes begin to secrete androgens. Androgens are the male hormones (such as testosterone) that cause the development of male sex characteristics such as facial hair. These hormones also stimulate other cells in the testicles to manufacture sperm. From puberty until sometime in old age, the continuous secretion of androgens results in a constant production of sperm.

After sperm have been formed, they move into the *epididymis*, the tube that coils along the back of each testicle, where they continue to develop. They are so tiny they cannot be seen without a microscope. The mature sperm is composed of an oval head that contains the chromosomes (the genetic material) and a long, whip-like tail that propels it with great vigor and speed. "Every one of them has an outboard motor, they know where they want to go, and there are millions of them," is the way a family planning expert recently described them. It takes a sperm about 72 days to grow to maturity, at which time it passes into another tube, the *vas deferens*, or sperm duct. Each vas runs from the epididymis up to the outside of the bladder. At this end the duct is wider and has enough space to store sperm in preparation for an ejaculation.

Just beneath the bladder lies the *prostate* gland, which produces secretions that help sperm survive after ejaculation. These secretions mix with the sperm after they leave the vas deferens. The mixture is called semen.

The *urethra*, the tube in which this mixing takes place, passes through the prostate, which enables the prostate secretions to enter the urethra through tiny ducts. The male urethra has two functions. When a man urinates, it transports urine from the bladder. During intercourse, it carries semen. When a man is sexually stimulated, the opening between the bladder and the urethra is closed to prevent urine from joining the semen. (After a man has been sexually aroused, it takes a short time for this system to reverse itself so he is able to urinate.)

At the peak of sexual excitement, the man's pelvic muscles tighten, forcing semen down the urethra and out the penis. This is called an orgasm, or ejaculating, or having a climax. Each ejaculate contains tens of millions of sperm—but only one actually gets to fertilize an egg.

THE FEMALE

If a woman is not familiar with her sexual anatomy, looking at the following illustration (Figure 1.3) may be helpful. However, looking at and touching your own anatomy may be an even better

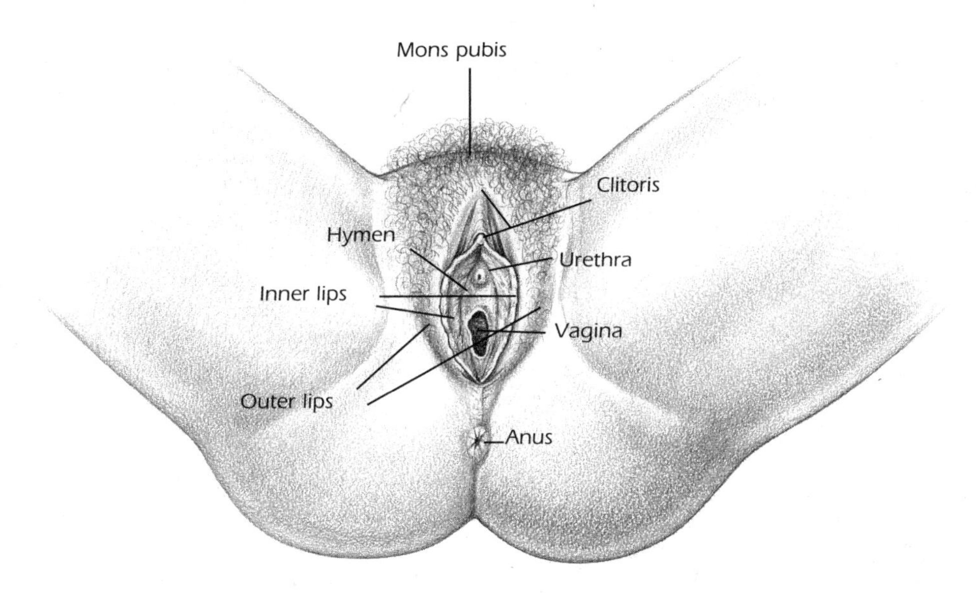

FIGURE 1.3 The Female Reproductive System (Exam View)

approach. You can use a mirror to see your external genitals if you wish, or you can rely on touch to determine where most of these structures are and how they feel. Being familiar with your body makes it easier to use birth control and may increase your pleasure during sex. If you want to insert a diaphragm, for instance, it is helpful to know just how long your vagina is and exactly where near its end your cervix lies.

The exterior sexual structures of the female are the mons pubis, the labia or "lips" of the vagina, the clitoris, the hymen, and the vaginal opening. The visible, exterior sexual structures together are called the vulva or external genitals.

The vagina leads to the internal reproductive organs: the cervix, the uterus, the fallopian tubes, and the ovaries. These lie inside the pelvis, supported and protected by the pelvic muscles and bones.

The *mons pubis* is the most noticeable part of the female genital area. It's the soft mound of fatty tissue below the belly that covers and protects the joining of the pubic bones, the pubic symphysis. During puberty, the mons becomes covered with hair that also covers the external genitals.

The opening to the vagina is protected by the *labia*. In some women, the *labia majora*, the outermost lips around the vaginal opening, are darker than the surrounding skin. The *labia minora* lie within the labia majora and are more delicate. They are sensitive to touch, and with sexual stimulation they become filled with blood and turn darker. The area of skin between the labia and the anus (the opening of the rectum) is the *perineum*, which often is also quite sensitive to stimulation.

The labia minora are joined at the front to form a soft fold of skin that looks like a little hood. This protects the *clitoris*, the most sensitive part of a woman's genitals. The clitoris contains many nerve endings which transmit sensory messages when the clitoris is touched, especially sexually. The clitoris has often been compared to the penis in its anatomy and reaction to stimulation. If you press the clitoris with your fingers, under its skin you can feel the firm but movable shaft that connects it to the pubic bones.

Between the clitoris and the vagina is a small opening for the *urethra*. As in males, the urethra is the tube that carries urine from the bladder.

In addition to being shielded by the labia, the vaginal opening in young girls may be partially covered by the *hymen*. This is a thin, usually stretchable tissue that is partially open to let menstrual blood flow through. In most women, the hymen opening is large enough to permit the use of tampons. When intercourse takes place, especially for the first time, the opening in the hymen often is stretched further by the penis. Sometimes it is pushed aside so hard it tears and may bleed a little.

The hymen varies a great deal from woman to woman and girl to girl in its flexibility and in the size of its opening. A woman who is sexually active may have a hymen that is still in one piece simply because it is very flexible. Or a woman with no sexual experience may have almost no hymen—just because that is the way her body developed.

The *vagina* is the passage that connects the external genitals to the cervix (Figure 1.4). Its length may vary from 2 1/2 to 4 inches. The vagina slants back slightly toward the spine. It is connected to the uterus at the cervix, which is the mouth of the uterus. Its muscu-

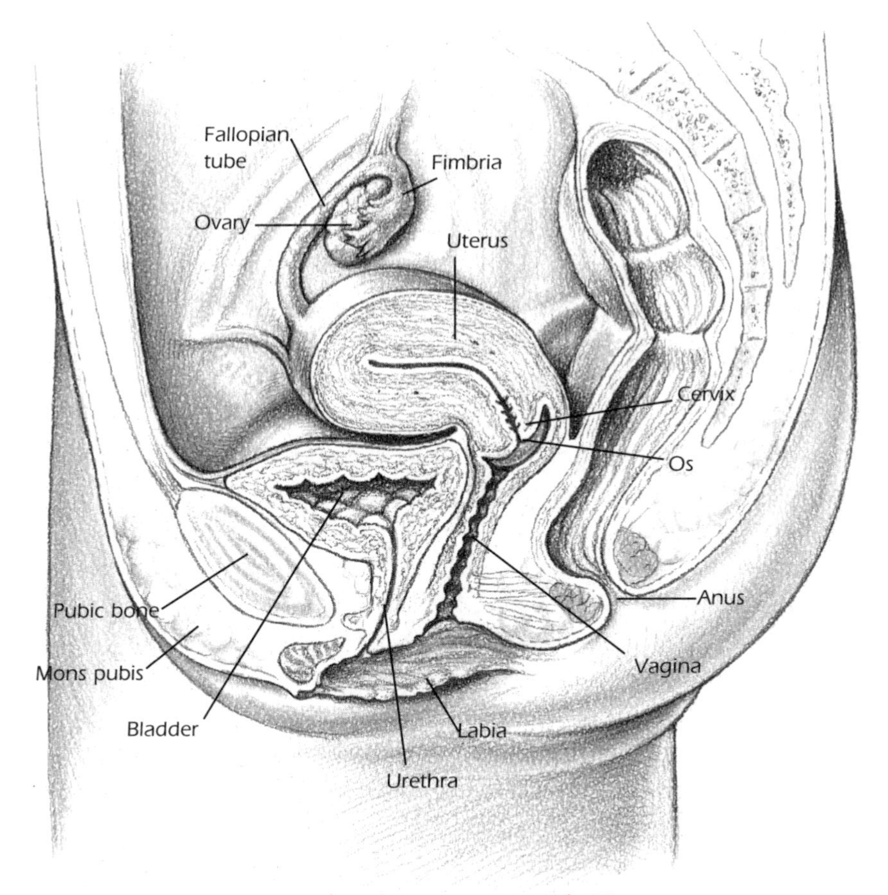

FIGURE 1.4 The Female Reproductive System (Side View)

lar walls are lined with a folded mucous membrane and contain many blood vessels. When you examine it with your fingers, the vagina feels both soft and muscular. In most women, the lower third is sensitive to sexual stimulation and the upper portion is less responsive. The vagina's walls are folded in on themselves so closely they touch, yet they have a great capacity for expanding around an object such as a penis, a baby, or a diaphragm. The mucous membrane lining the vagina can change from almost dry to very wet because it secretes fluids, particularly around the time of ovulation, during pregnancy, and when the woman is sexually aroused.

The *uterus* resembles an upside-down pear about the size of a fist. The lower, narrow end of the uterus, or *cervix*, extends down into the vagina and has an opening called the *os*. The tip of the cervix is small and firm and feels like the tip of a nose. Before a woman has a child, the os is very small—about the diameter of a straw. The cervix and uterus have thick, muscular, very flexible walls designed to accommodate a fetus and the effort of childbirth.

Glands in the cervix secrete mucus that varies both in amount and consistency during the course of the month, depending on the levels of estrogen and progesterone, the hormones produced by the woman's body. When progesterone levels are high, for example, the cervix secretes a thick, nonstretchable mucus that effectively plugs the os against the entrance of sperm. During ovulation, however, estrogen levels are high and the mucus becomes thin and stretchy and is hospitable to sperm.

The cervix shifts position during the menstrual cycle, making it easier to reach on some days. A few days before ovulation it is high in the vagina and then, just before menstruation, it is lower. The os also changes throughout the cycle, opening wider before ovulation and before menstruation.

Sperm deposited inside the vagina or *just outside it* quickly propel themselves up into the os, through the uterus, and into the fallopian tubes, where fertilization takes place if an egg is waiting (Figure 1.5). How easily sperm move from the vagina and through the cervix depends on the type of cervical mucus present. The mucus produced near the time of ovulation protects sperm from the acid environment of the vagina and assists their progress toward the fallopian tubes.

After fertilization, the egg cell begins the process of dividing as it moves through the fallopian tubes and into the uterus. There it implants itself in the *endometrium*, or uterine lining, in order to continue developing into an embryo and then a fetus. When the fetus is fully developed, the muscular walls of the uterus will produce strong contractions to push it down through the cervix and vagina, which stretch to permit the passage of the baby.

In most women the uterus is slanted, with its top pointed toward the upper abdomen and the cervix aimed at the lower back. In some women, this angle is reversed and the cervix points forward, a differ-

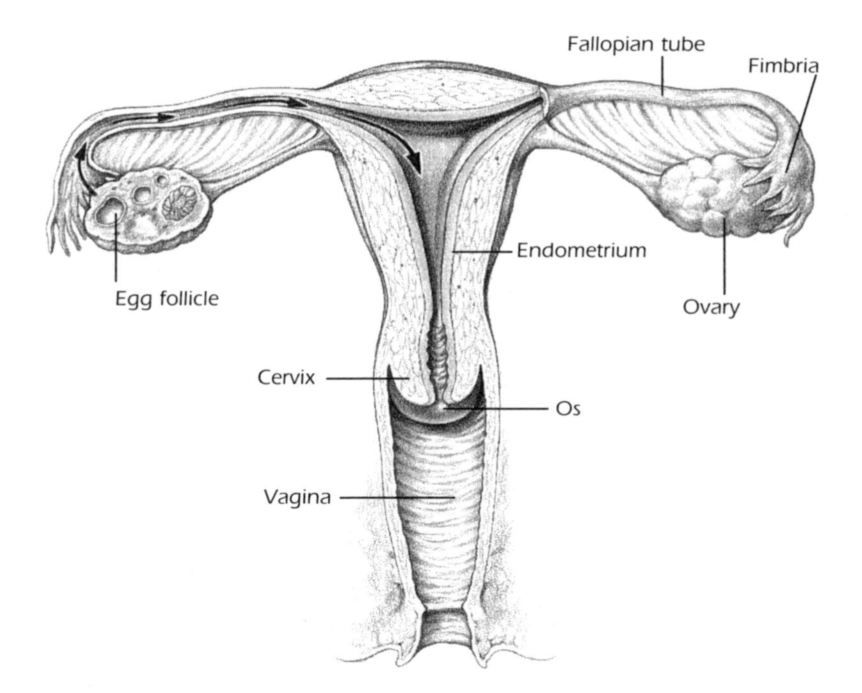

FIGURE 1.5 The Female Reproductive System (Frontal View)

ence that generally does not affect pregnancy or childbirth but can affect your choice of contraceptive. A forward tilt to the cervix may make the cervical cap or diaphragm less reliable because the forward slant can allow these devices to be easily dislodged during intercourse.

On each side of the uterus is a slender, delicate *fallopian tube*, which is three to four inches long. The end of each tube is shaped somewhat like a funnel with fringed ends, called the fimbria, that almost touch the ovary. The ovaries are small, oval shaped, and about the size of walnuts. There is one near each fallopian tube. They contain thousands of tiny egg follicles that hold a lifetime supply of undeveloped egg cells. The ovaries also produce the hormones needed for reproduction. When an egg matures, it is expelled from the ovary and the fimbria gather it into the fallopian tube. The walls of the fallopian tubes are lined with fine, hair-like projections called cilia. The cilia and muscular contractions of the tube move the egg along to the uterus.

OVULATION

At the time a baby girl is born, her two ovaries already contain all the egg cells she might ever need. Of the million or so eggs in her ovaries, only about 300 to 500 will actually be released (ovulated) during the years between puberty and menopause.

As a girl approaches puberty, her body steps up the production of the hormones that permit ovulation and reproduction. The most important hormones are estrogen, progesterone, follicle-stimulating hormone (FSH), luteinizing hormone (LH), and gonadotropin-releasing hormone (GnRH). The production of each of these hormones increases and decreases in a regular pattern every month. During this cycle, changes in hormone levels cause an egg in one ovary to mature. Each egg develops within a follicle, a hollow, fluid-filled sphere of cells. When an egg is ready for fertilization, the follicle breaks open and the egg floats out and normally is captured by the fimbria. Usually only one egg cell develops each month; if two eggs mature and both are fertilized successfully, the result is fraternal twins. (Identical twins result when one fertilized egg cell divides into two.)

Ovulation usually takes place approximately halfway between menstrual periods, most commonly 14 days *before* the next menstrual period, although this can vary greatly from woman to woman and from month to month (see Chapter 14 on cycle-based fertility control). While the egg is maturing, the increased levels of hormones cause the lining of the uterus to prepare for nurturing a fertilized egg.

Physical and emotional events can have a considerable effect on hormone production and changes in hormone levels can alter the menstrual cycle; as a result, ovulation can occur at an unexpected time. In some instances, ovulation has been known to take place even during menstruation.

Some experts believe that sperm can survive in the reproductive tract for up to 7 days, and an egg cell can be fertilized anytime during the 24 hours after it has left the ovary. No one knows precisely how long eggs and sperm live in the human reproductive system and, therefore, fertilization is considered possible for about an 8-day span in each menstrual cycle. If an egg is unfertilized, it simply is absorbed by the uterus or flushed out with the menstrual blood.

FERTILIZATION

In order to be fertilized, the egg must be penetrated by a single sperm. Although each ejaculate contains millions of sperm, usually only a few hundred reach the fallopian tubes, a journey that takes healthy sperm only a few minutes. If ovulation has recently occurred, the sperm will encounter an egg cell ready for fertilization. Egg cells are covered by a thick, tough, transparent layer called the zona pellucida, which functions as a sophisticated biological security system. The zona pellucida chemically controls the entry of sperm into the egg. Although there may be hundreds of tail-lashing sperm clustered around the egg, only one actually succeeds in penetrating that outer layer. As soon as it does, a chemical reaction automatically shuts out the rest. This reaction prevents the genetic confusion that would occur if the chromosomes of more than one sperm combined with the chromosomes of the egg.

When fertilization takes place, the genetic materials from the sperm and egg combine, and the egg cell begins to divide. While the egg is in the fallopian tube, there is a considerable risk that it may fail to develop. If it survives, it continues to divide, and by the time it reaches the uterus it is a cluster of cells the size of a speck of dust. By the sixth or seventh day after ovulation, the cluster begins to embed itself in the lining of the uterus, which has become thick, soft, and engorged with blood in preparation for nurturing an embryo. The egg cells continue to divide and by the eighteenth day after fertilization the cells that are destined to form the spinal cord can be detected. At this point the cluster of cells can be called a true embryo.

TUBAL (ECTOPIC) PREGNANCY

If the fallopian tube is abnormal in some way or damaged from pelvic inflammatory disease, the fertilized egg may not be able to travel through the tube to the uterus. Instead, it may start to grow in the fallopian tube, and the resulting pregnancy is called tubal, or ectopic. ("Ectopic" means "out of place.") Because fallopian tubes are not designed to sustain a pregnancy, the growing embryo usually ruptures or otherwise damages the tube and the tissues around it, causing severe abdominal pain and vaginal bleeding. Tubal pregnancies can be a life-threatening problem, requiring surgery to remove the embryo and to repair, if possible, the torn or scarred tissue. In the United States, about 1 in 100 pregnancies is ectopic, probably because of the relatively high rates of STDs and the pelvic inflammation that follows STDs.

MENSTRUATION

If fertilization does not take place and no cluster of egg cells is implanted in the uterus, the production of hormones declines and the blood-filled endometrium, no longer needed to nourish a possible embryo, breaks up. Over several days it is expelled from the uterus, sometimes with the help of contractions that may range from mild to painful. This shedding of tissue and blood is called menstruation, or a monthly period. The monthly sequence of events is called the menstrual cycle and its sole purpose is to prepare your body for a probable pregnancy.

This cycle of events occurs every month unless an egg is fertilized and successfully attaches to the uterus lining. When such an attachment takes place, the lining is not expelled, there is no menstrual bleeding, and a pregnancy is under way.

SEXUAL INTERCOURSE

When a woman becomes sexually aroused, a cascade of changes takes place throughout her body. Blood flow to the genital area increases, and her clitoris swells, becomes erect, and sometimes is so sensitive it hurts when it is touched. The labia minora swell and deepen in color, the vagina becomes moist, and its opening widens. The entire genital area seems to increase in sensitivity. In addition, the breasts swell and the nipples become erect. The woman's heart rate speeds up, she breathes faster and harder, and her muscles tighten. If sexual stimulation continues, arousal intensifies and leads to an orgasm. During orgasm, the muscles around the vagina, uterus, and rectum contract once or several times and then release. Afterwards, the process slowly begins to reverse. Muscles relax, blood flows out of the swollen tissues, and the clitoris and vagina return to their usual size.

When a man is sexually stimulated, his body undergoes many of the same physical changes. As we mentioned earlier, his penis becomes erect as blood flows into its tissues and stays there because the valves of the penile blood system have closed. His pelvic muscles tighten and force semen from the prostate and epididymis into the urethra. If stimulation continues, it triggers ejaculation. Afterward, his muscles relax, the valves in the blood vessels open, the blood drains away, and the penis becomes soft again.

After orgasm, most men experience an interval in which they have no physical response to further sexual stimulation. Women may or may not feel this same relaxation. Some women, if stimulation continues, experience multiple orgasms.

HOW CONTRACEPTION WORKS

The various methods of birth control function at different points in the reproductive process. They either suppress ovulation entirely, stop the sperm and egg from meeting in the fallopian tubes, or create an environment hostile to fertilization and implantation.

- Barrier contraceptives such as condoms, the diaphragm, and the cervical cap physically block sperm from entering the cervix.
- The chemical spermicide in creams, jellies, foams, vaginal suppositories, and contraceptive film kills sperm upon contact.
- Birth control pills, Depo-Provera, and Norplant implants alter the normal levels of the hormones estrogen and progesterone in

women. Pills combining small amounts of the synthetic forms of both hormones suppress ovulation. Norplant and pills containing only a synthetic progesterone-like hormone may also suppress ovulation but not consistently. These single-hormone methods thicken the cervical mucus to make it impervious to sperm. They also hinder the normal monthly changes in the lining of the uterus.

- Intrauterine devices (IUDs) with copper work by reducing the number and viability of sperm reaching the egg and by impeding the movement of the egg into the uterus.
- Sterilization is surgery to block the woman's fallopian or the man's vas deferens tubes, preventing egg and sperm from uniting.
- Fertility awareness methods teach a woman how to know when she is fertile. During her fertile days she and her partner either abstain from sex or use a barrier contraceptive.
- If unprotected intercourse takes place during a time a woman might be fertile, an emergency contraception method can prevent implantation if it is used soon after that intercourse (see Chapter 16 on emergency contraception).
- Abortion ends a pregnancy either via a suction procedure during the first 12 weeks (first trimester) or, in the second trimester, by using dilation and evacuation (D&E). Medical abortions that depend on a combination of drugs are becoming available for early first trimester abortions.

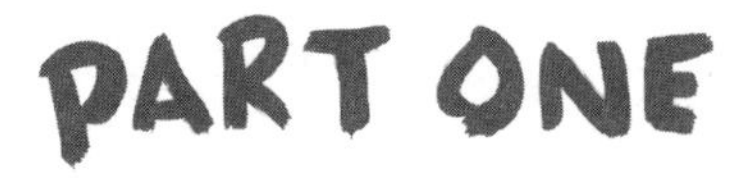

Barrier Methods

2

The Male Condom

The male condom is a soft, flexible cover that fits over the penis. It may be made of latex, polyurethane, Tactylon, or treated animal tissue that is thin, strong, and flexible. (The female condom is described in Chapter 3.) Because a condom prevents semen from entering the vagina, it is a very effective barrier to pregnancy. Except for those made of animal skin, condoms also act as a barrier to viruses and bacteria, protecting *both* partners from sexually transmitted diseases such as syphilis, chlamydia, gonorrhea, genital warts, genital herpes, candidiasis, trichomoniasis, and AIDS. Some of these diseases may make you very sick—and some can make you infertile.

Unless you are in a mutually monogamous, long-term relationship, you use a condom not only to protect against pregnancy, but because it is possible for *any* sexually active person to have an STD and not know it. Many STDs have no symptoms, especially in the early stages. It is simply common sense to protect yourself and your partner.

Next to abstinence, condoms are the best protection against AIDS, a fatal disease that today is the number one killer of U.S. men aged 25 to 44 and the third leading killer of U.S. women aged 25 and 44. The majority of people who have AIDS were infected through sex, and many men and women who die of AIDS in their twenties were infected during their teens. Today it is a disease of heterosexuals as well as homosexuals.

To improve their effectiveness as well as prevent STDs, condoms can be used with a spermicide—a sperm-killing jelly or cream.

Condoms are easy to use and do not require a physical exam or a doctor's prescription. Furthermore, they are available in small packages that can be tucked into a pocket or purse or stored in a bedside table or bathroom cabinet. They are sold in many types of stores and at health centers. Individually they cost very little, but if they are used often, the cost can add up.

It is not unusual today for women who use other birth control methods like the Pill or Depo-Provera, or men who have had a vasectomy, to use a condom as well—for protection against STDs, including AIDS. To protect against infection, condoms should be used for oral and anal sex as well as vaginal intercourse.

Male condoms are available in dozens of brands and models, ranging from plain to those that come in different thicknesses, textures, and colors. Condoms that are slightly thicker are less likely to break than thinner ones. Those with a reservoir tip also may be less likely to break or overflow when filled with semen. Some are coated with a lubricant or a spermicide.

Both latex and lambskin condoms are available in several shapes: tapered, flared, or contoured for a tighter fit. Polyurethane and Tactylon condoms are so new they are currently available in only one shape and are either lubricated or plain. Because so many brands and styles are available, the best way to find the type that works best for you is by trying various kinds.

Condoms are usually made in the same basic shape. Most measure between 6 and 8 inches long and are approximately 2 inches in diameter. Because they generally are so flexible, and an exact fit is unnecessary, most condoms are not sold by size. Several brands, however, do offer a large size. If a condom seems too loose or too tight, or you are having problems with it slipping off, try other types or brands until you get a fit you like. Most condoms are not expensive, and it is worth experimenting with different ones if it makes a difference in how you feel about using them.

IN A NUTSHELL

THE MALE CONDOM

The male condom is a birth control method used by a man. He puts it on his penis before having sex. It catches the sperm when he "comes" (ejaculates) so the sperm does not go into the woman's body. Latex and polyurethane condoms not only prevent pregnancy, they also are the best protection against STDs, including AIDS.

Condoms are not very expensive. You can buy them at a drugstore or large discount store without anyone asking questions. You do not need to be a certain age or have a prescription. Some health centers and clinics will give you condoms for free.

You should remember not to touch a latex condom with anything greasy because oil weakens the rubber and the condom might break. You can buy special creams or, even better, use a spermicidal foam or gel with a condom. Condoms do not break often but for extra protection, in case one does, the woman can also put spermicide (a sperm-killing product) into her vagina before having sex.

To protect yourself and your partner, you must use a latex or polyurethane condom every time you have sex.

CONDOMS AND SEXUAL PLEASURE

Although some men complain that wearing a condom diminishes their pleasure, others find that a small decrease in stimulation allows them to prolong their sexual play because they stay hard longer. This seldom-mentioned aspect of condoms is particularly useful if you are easily aroused or ejaculate prematurely.

Almost half the condoms sold today are bought by girls and women. Instead of thinking of the condom as an unwelcome interruption, many savvy couples make the act of putting the condom on the penis a part of their lovemaking. In fact, a recent survey discovered that, in many cases, both partners found it sexually stimulating.

LATEX CONDOMS

Latex condoms are readily available and are the least expensive. Extra thin latex condoms may permit more sensation, but they also tear more easily and must be handled carefully. It is worthwhile noting that some condoms that are advertised as "thin" are not truly thinner, and some latex condoms promoted as "stronger" proved not to be as sturdy as others when they were tested by Consumers Union. The laboratory test results of many brands of condoms were published in the May 1995 issue of *Consumer Reports* magazine.

Latex condoms that glow in the dark, are flavored, or are brightly colored may not be as protective as plain, ordinary condoms. The flavoring or coloring process may have a negative effect on the quality of the latex. If you are interested in using them, read the labels carefully for information about protection against disease and pregnancy. Many are sold as novelties and are not for use to prevent pregnancy or disease.

ALLERGIC EFFECTS

Allergy to products made of latex is on the rise, particularly among people who must use rubber gloves or other latex products. Because allergies build up over time, and there are so many latex products used today, experts are expecting more people to develop this allergy.

The most common form of the allergy is like the reaction to poison ivy—the skin turns red and swells anytime up to 2 days after exposure to a latex product, including a condom. Allergic reactions that occur *immediately* after contact with latex or spermicide can be more serious and require medical treatment. Fortunately, such reactions are rare.

Either partner can have an allergic reaction to condoms, and the cause may not always be the latex. There also can be a reaction to the spermicide or the lubricant that coats some condoms. Sometimes a perfume in the spermicide or lubricant is the culprit. Switching to another brand of condom may prevent this type of reaction. If that does not work, then the active ingredient in the spermicide, nonoxynol-9, may be the cause. Spermicide allergy can be averted by using plain condoms with no spermicide coating.

If you suspect that the latex is the source of your irritation, you can try other brands of latex condoms—in the hope of finding a better manufactured latex—or else move to the new nonlatex condoms that are now available.

POLYURETHANE CONDOMS

New to the market are condoms made of a thin, clear, soft polyurethane. They recently have been approved for sale by the FDA, mostly for people who are sensitive to latex and cannot use latex condoms. Polyurethane condoms are too new to have been included in any long-term studies of condom effectiveness in actual use. Laboratory tests, however, have shown that sperm, viruses, and bacteria cannot pass through this material.

Because they are thin and transparent, polyurethane condoms may be more comfortable to use. In addition, polyurethane transfers body heat more readily, so there is more sensation during sex. In a survey of users, more than half the men and women who tried these new condoms said they liked them better than latex. Polyurethane condoms are sold in most large drugstore chains under the brand name "Avanti."

TACTYLON CONDOMS

Another new, nonlatex condom is made of a material called *Tactylon*, a thermoplastic polymer. Like latex and polyurethane, in lab tests Tactylon did not permit the passage of sperm, viruses, or bacteria, and should provide good protection against disease.

Tactylon condoms are very thin, soft, strong, and extremely stretchy. They allow greater sensitivity during use than do latex condoms. They also tend to maintain their strength and are not easily degraded by temperature, sunlight, or other storage conditions that reduce the durability of latex condoms. In addition, Tactylon is not damaged by oils.

Tactylon condoms will reach drugstores in early 1998. The brand name that will be used has not yet been decided; however, the condoms will be identified on the package as being made of Tactylon.

"SKIN" CONDOMS

Skin condoms are made from treated lamb membranes. They are thinner and stronger than latex, and some men believe they permit more sensation. Because they are not made from latex, they are an option for men and women who are allergic to that rubber product. *Skin condoms, however, do not protect against diseases.* The membrane has tiny pores that are too small for sperm to get through but are large enough to allow the passage of the viruses and bacteria that cause STDs, including AIDS. The U.S. Food and Drug Administration (FDA) does not allow skin condoms to be labeled as protection against sexually transmitted diseases.

EFFECTIVENESS

Studies of actual condom use reveal a failure rate that ranges from 3 to 12 percent. In other words, 3 to 12 pregnancies can be expected among every 100 women whose partners use condoms for 1 year. For birth control, condoms are more protective in typical use than a diaphragm but less effective than the Pill. They may offer greater protection from pregnancy and from disease if they are used with a spermicide. As with most contraceptives, the greatest number of condom failures occur during the first year of use. Experience in using a condom reduces the likelihood of it slipping or breaking. Condoms that have been stored for a long while are more likely to break than condoms that were manufactured recently. Check the expiration date before you buy, and avoid old condoms.

As with any birth control method, effectiveness also depends a great deal on how committed the users are to preventing pregnancy. Obviously, couples who use a condom perfectly and use it every time they have sex will have the fewest failures. Using a spermicide plus a condom may improve the condom's effectiveness in preventing both pregnancy and disease. When used in anal sex, however, a condom is more likely to break and slip than when used for vaginal sex, although these problems still occur infrequently.

The FDA regulates condoms as medical devices and sends inspectors unannounced to factories to test condoms with an air-burst test: condoms are inflated until they pop and a computer records the air pressure they withstand. The amount of air pressure a condom can take indicates its strength and flexibility. This allows inspectors to test samples from a production run and from their performance

WHO SHOULD NOT DEPEND ON CONDOMS?

Condoms may not be the best birth control method for you if (1) you tend to forget to keep a supply on hand, (2) you are inclined to skip using protection "just this once," or (3) you or your partner are still embarrassed or uncomfortable using condoms after you have tried them several times.

(It is worth making an extra effort to learn to use and become comfortable with this method, however, because a condom is the best disease protection available.)

estimate the failure rate for the entire lot. (Do not test a condom yourself by filling it with water or air before you use it. You will weaken it.)

USING A CONDOM

- Do not tear the package open with your teeth—you could tear the condom as well.
- If condoms are new to you, it is a really good idea to practice putting one on before you need it. You can practice on an erect penis or on cylinder-shaped objects such as a slim cucumber or banana. (Throw out the practice condoms.)
- A condom comes rolled up in a package. For it to work right, it must be unrolled *all* the way up the erect penis (Figure 2.1). If you are not circumcised, pull back the foreskin before putting on the condom. If the condom does not unroll easily, you may be doing it backwards. The rolled-up rim should always be on the outside of the condom.
- If you have unrolled the condom the wrong way, do not try to use it. Throw it away and start over with a new one.
- If the brand you are using does not have a reservoir tip (it will say so on the package), grasp about half an inch of the condom's tip between two fingers while you roll it on with the other hand. This makes sure there is room at the tip for semen and lessens the chance that the condom will be stressed and break or overflow when it is full. You will also be pinching out any air at the tip, which helps

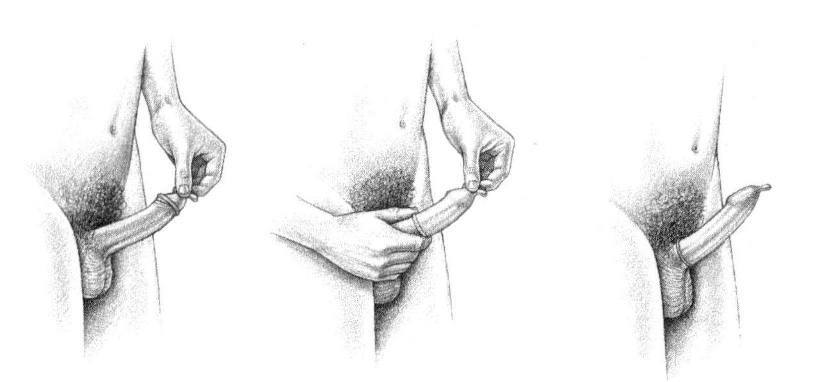

FIGURE 2.1 How to Use a Condom

keep the condom from breaking. And as you handle a condom, be careful not to tear it with your fingernails or rings.

- Until the condom is securely in place, keep the penis away from the vagina—drops of semen may leak from the penis before ejaculation and can cause pregnancy or carry HIV.
- Keep at least one or two extra condoms with you for backup.

Use a new condom every time you have sex. This is the most important rule in the successful use of condoms. The average man produces millions of healthy, active sperm every day, and the supply is seldom diminished by frequent ejaculations. No matter how many times you have sex, even during a fairly short period of time, use a new condom each time. And use a condom for oral and anal sex—STDs can be transmitted via the mouth or anus.

Do not begin intercourse until the vagina is well lubricated. When a woman is sexually aroused, the vagina naturally lubricates. Without this slipperiness to help the penis slide in, the condom can tear. If you are using a latex condom and want more lubrication, use water, the spermicidal cream or gel made for diaphragms, or a *water-based* lubricating jelly such as K-Y Jelly, Women's Health Institute Lubricating Gel, or the lubricating jelly of any major drugstore brand. They are sold in the feminine hygiene or family planning section of drugstores. The packages usually say they are oil free and made to be used with a diaphragm or condom. If you are in doubt about any product, the list of ingredients on the package indicates whether it contains any oil.

If the condom starts to slip off, stop and check it. Replace it with a new one if necessary and think about buying a different brand next time.

After climax (ejaculation or coming), withdraw your penis while it is still erect, or the condom will slip off and sperm will spill out. Pull the penis and the condom slowly from the vagina while holding the rim of the condom against the base of the penis. Look at the condom for signs of a leak.

Remove it carefully, away from your partner's genital area. Wrap it in a tissue and throw it away.

If the condom breaks, slips, or leaks, there are a couple of things you can do to prevent pregnancy. If you have spermicide handy, immediately insert an applicator full of it well up into the vagina if you did not do so earlier. This is not a guarantee against pregnancy or infection, but it does provide some protection nevertheless. As soon as possible, talk to your nearest family planning clinic or your doctor about emergency contraception. Emergency contraception is simply the use of conventional contraceptive pills in high doses within 72 hours after intercourse. It is safe and effective but needs to be prescribed by a health care professional. (For more information on emergency contraception, see Chapter 16.)

Oils and grease are dangerous to latex condoms. When oils, oil-based lotions, or greasy hands touch latex they react with the rubber and weaken it. Then the condom is more likely to rip during use or develop tiny holes you may not see. Keep baby oils, hand lotions, face creams, ointments, petroleum jelly, massage oil, grease, or butter away from condoms and other latex contraceptives such as diaphragms or cervical caps. Even grease from french fries or makeup can damage latex, so both partners should wash their hands before touching a condom.

For additional protection, before intercourse, insert into the vagina an applicator of spermicidal foam, jelly, or gel made to be used with a diaphragm or a contraceptive film. Although some condoms are pretreated with a similar spermicide, there may not be enough to offer adequate protection. Spermicide use is an especially good idea during the most fertile time in the menstrual cycle. If either of you is allergic to spermicide, however, you can use the condom alone.

CARE AND STORAGE

Condoms can last for several years if they are kept sealed in their packages and stored away from light and heat. The refrigerator is a good place to keep condoms—and any other latex rubber contraceptive—especially in hot weather. Condoms deteriorate fast if kept in the glove compartment of a car, for instance, or in a purse or coat that is hung in a warm closet or left for a while in the sun or over a radiator. Condoms can also weaken if they are exposed to body heat for some time by being carried in an inside pocket.

If you have been carrying a condom around with you for several months, particularly in the summer, throw it out and replace it with a new one. This is especially important if you carry a condom in your wallet, because it is exposed to a lot of mechanical stress as well. The cost of a new package is a small price to pay for good protection. And do not remove the condom from its sealed packet until you are ready to use it.

COST

You can get latex condoms for as little as three for $2.50 (about 84 cents each) at large chain drugstores or discount stores. Buying in large quantities, however, is by far the best approach—some brands offer 36 latex condoms for $18.99, which brings the cost to just over 50 cents each. Nonlatex condoms are more expensive—they currently sell at three for $6.00 and six for $10.50 at large drugstore chains. Lambskin condoms are the most expensive: three for $12.00 and twelve for $35.00 are typical prices.

Although the price for a single condom or even one package may seem low, if they are used many times a week, month after month, the cost is similar to that of the Pill. Condoms are not covered by insurance. Over the long term, the IUD or the Pill would be much cheaper and more likely to be paid for by insurance or Medicaid; however, these methods do not protect against STDs. Today, for the best protection, many couples use condoms plus a second method.

3

The Female Condom

Currently, there is only one version of a female condom on the market: the Reality Female Condom. It is a soft, loose-fitting tube or long pouch that is made of a very thin, strong, transparent polyurethane, approximately 3 inches in diameter and 6 to 7 inches long. It looks a bit like a miniature wind sock (Figure 3.1). It is designed to line the inner contours of the vagina and protect a woman against sperm and the bacteria and viruses that cause disease, including AIDS. The female condom has a flexible, narrow ring at both ends. The slightly smaller ring inside the closed end helps to place that end over the cervix and to hold it there. The ring at the open end remains outside the vagina and serves as the entry for the penis. The pouch is lubricated both inside and out. Like the male condom, it is meant for one-time use.

The female condom not only protects the vagina and cervix from sperm and microbes, it is sized so that the open end also covers a woman's external genitals and the base of her partner's penis, offering both of them excellent protection against disease.

Because it is made of polyurethane, the female condom has the advantage of being stronger than latex and less likely to tear or develop tiny holes. It will not aggravate a latex allergy. It is not

IN A NUTSHELL

THE FEMALE CONDOM

The female condom is larger and looser than the male condom. The closed end fits over the cervix, inside the vagina. The open end hangs slightly outside and protects the lips of the vagina. Because it is made of polyurethane, it becomes very soft and flexible when it is in place. It is very effective in protecting both partners against pregnancy and diseases, including AIDS.

Like a male condom, the female condom can be bought by anyone. You do not need a prescription. It is sold in drugstores under the name Reality Female Condom. The cost is higher than a male condom.

You will want to practice putting it in place before you use it. It does not interrupt lovemaking because you can insert it ahead of time.

Although the female condom looks a little strange, many women and men find they like it. A man likes it because it's more comfortable than a male condom and he doesn't have to pull out as soon as he has come (ejaculated). Women like it because it gives them control over their own safety.

affected by oil-based creams or lotions and is less vulnerable to deterioration caused by exposure to heat or lengthy storage. Like the Avanti condom, it transfers body heat easily, which means it quickly feels warm and soft and permits more sensation.

When it was tested in actual use, about one-third of the men said they preferred the female condom over the male condom because it was roomier. Some men noted that it felt more natural to them because the penis could move freely in and out. They liked the fact that they did not have to interrupt their lovemaking to put on a condom. They also could linger as long as they wanted after ejaculation because, unlike using a male condom, they did not have to withdraw while their penis was still erect. You can put the female condom in place up to 8 hours before intercourse and you do not need a spermicide for extra safety. The female condom should be removed before you stand up.

For many women, however, the major advantage of the female condom is that it gives them control over their own protection against STDs, instead of trying to convince their partners to protect them by using a condom.

The female condom can be

WHO LIKES THE FEMALE CONDOM?

- Women who are concerned about STD transmission and cannot get a man to use a condom.
- Women who prefer to have control over risks in their lives.
- Women who have sexual relationships with more than one partner or have one monogamous relationship after another.
- Women who use oral contraceptives, Depo-Provera, Norplant, or an IUD but also want protection against STDs.
- Women interested in trying different barrier methods.

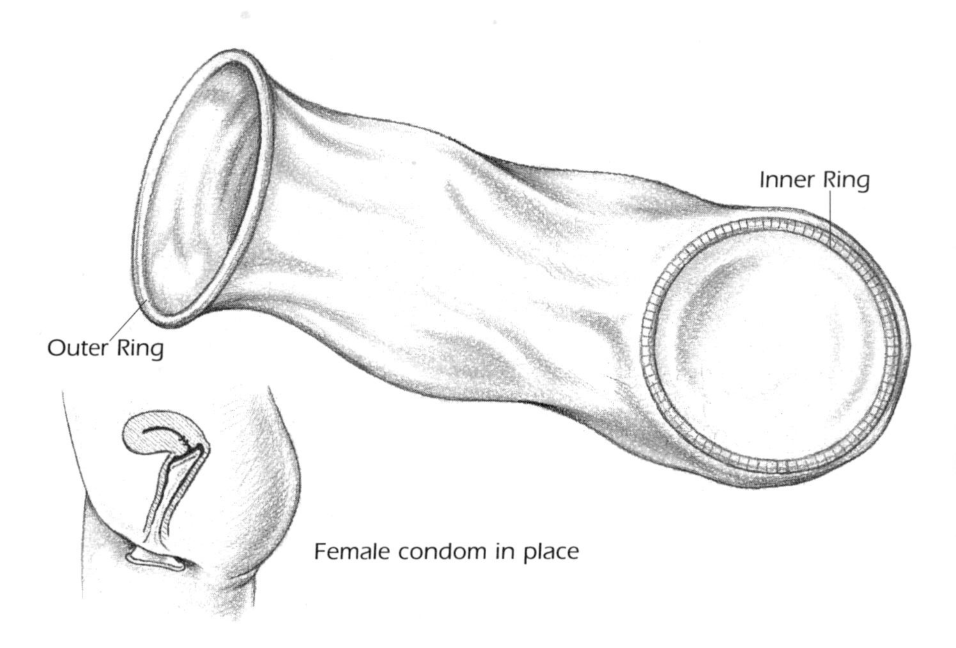

FIGURE 3.1 The Female Condom

bought without a prescription and at most drugstores. The package, while not as compact as packets of men's condoms, is small enough to tuck into a purse or pocket.

The female condom does not require a physical examination and a fitting like a diaphragm because it does not have to provide a snug cover for the cervix. It is protective because all the semen is trapped in its long pouch. However, if you have never used a barrier contraceptive like the diaphragm you may want to seek the help of a health care provider at a women's health center or family planning clinic.

Women's health clinics that offer the female condom report that their clients "either love it or hate it." In studies of the Reality condom, the women who used it said that the biggest disadvantage was the sensation of having something outside the vagina; however, many of those who used this type of condom for a week or two said they soon became accustomed to this and barely noticed it. Some found that the part of the condom that lies outside the body tended to stimulate the clitoris, adding to their pleasure. Although many of their partners reported that they could feel the condom, they did not necessarily find it objectionable.

The Reality condom can be noisy if the lubricant inside is not spread evenly around the outer end or if there just is not enough lubricant. Furthermore, if lovemaking is lengthy, the lubrication may get used up and the polyurethane will become somewhat dry. The solution is to add two drops (or more as needed) of lubricant to the entrance of the condom or on the penis. Extra lubricant is supplied with each starter package of Reality condoms.

EFFECTIVENESS

Laboratory tests of the polyurethane used in the Reality condom (and in the Avanti male condom) have demonstrated that the AIDS and hepatitis B viruses are not able to penetrate the polyurethane. (Hepatitis B is the smallest virus known to cause an STD.)

A study of the contraceptive effectiveness of the female condom in actual use found that it is as good as other barrier methods—the male condom, the diaphragm, or the cervical cap—in protecting against pregnancy. The rate of accidental pregnancy during a 6-month period ranged from 2.6 percent (for women who used the condom correctly and for every single intercourse) to 12.4 percent (for typical, less-than-perfect use). To arrive at a 12-month failure rate, the FDA doubled the rates from the 6-month study: the failure rate for perfect users is now listed as 5 percent and, for typical users, as 21 percent.

The results of this clinical study of effectiveness have led researchers to suggest that the *perfect* use of this condom could also substantially reduce women's risk of acquiring HIV. They estimate that, among women who have intercourse twice a week with an infected man, the annual risk of acquiring the infection could be reduced by 90 percent.

HEALTH EFFECTS

Because it is made of polyurethane rather than latex, the Reality condom is a good choice for the numbers of women (or their partners) who are allergic to latex rubber. In addition, it does not require the use of a spermicide, so it is attractive to those who are irritated by the ingredients in today's spermicides.

Although polyurethane is not as likely as latex to irritate the vagina or the penis, there is always a slight possibility that such irritations might occur. Frequent use of polyurethane condoms may sensitize some individuals to the material although, so far, this complaint has been rare. The symptoms are itching and mild pain.

USING A FEMALE CONDOM

Female condoms are available chiefly from large drugstore chains, where they are usually stocked near the supply of male condoms. They also can be bought at many women's health clinics.

Because the female condom is so new and looks so different, even someone who has used a diaphragm or a tampon may be nervous about trying it. It helps to have a sense of humor when trying it and to practice with it a few times before actually having sex. Take your time and become at ease with this type of condom before actually using it for protection.

Inserting the Female Condom

Before you try to insert the condom, read the section on female anatomy in Chapter 1 and familiarize yourself with your vagina and the location of your pubic bone and cervix. You will be much more relaxed about using any barrier contraceptive—and about sex—if you are acquainted with your own body.

Although the directions for inserting this condom are lengthy because they cover every detail, after a little practice you will find that insertion is quite simple and quick (Figure 3.2). If you have difficulty with it, take a break, relax, and re-read the directions given here or those that come with the package before you try again. Being relaxed and willing to experiment will make the process much easier.

- The closed end of the female condom is designed to fit over the cervix, and the open end stays on the outside of your body.
- The condom can be inserted anytime up to 8 hours before having sex.
- If you are not familiar with your vagina, check it out before you try inserting the condom. Use your middle finger to find your cervix at the upper end. It feels somewhat like the end of your nose, and it is about 3 inches from the vagina's opening. The vagina itself is not very long.
- To be sure the lubrication is spread evenly on the inside of the long pouch, from bottom to top, rub the outside of the condom gently. The lubricant is designed to make the inside of the condom feel similar to the naturally lubricated vagina. If the penis does not slip in and out easily during use, you can add more lubricant from the extra supply in the package.
- Before you try inserting the female condom, find a comfortable position. You can sit on the edge of a chair with your knees apart, or sit on the toilet, or lie down.
- Be sure the inside ring is down at the closed end of the tube. The inside ring is a bit smaller and thicker than the outside ring.
- To make it easier to insert the condom, add a drop or two of extra lubricant to the *outside* of the closed end of the pouch. Too much lubricant, however, may make it hard to grasp the ring firmly.
- Hold the pouch by the inside ring, with the open end hanging down. Squeeze the sides of the inner ring together to make it narrow

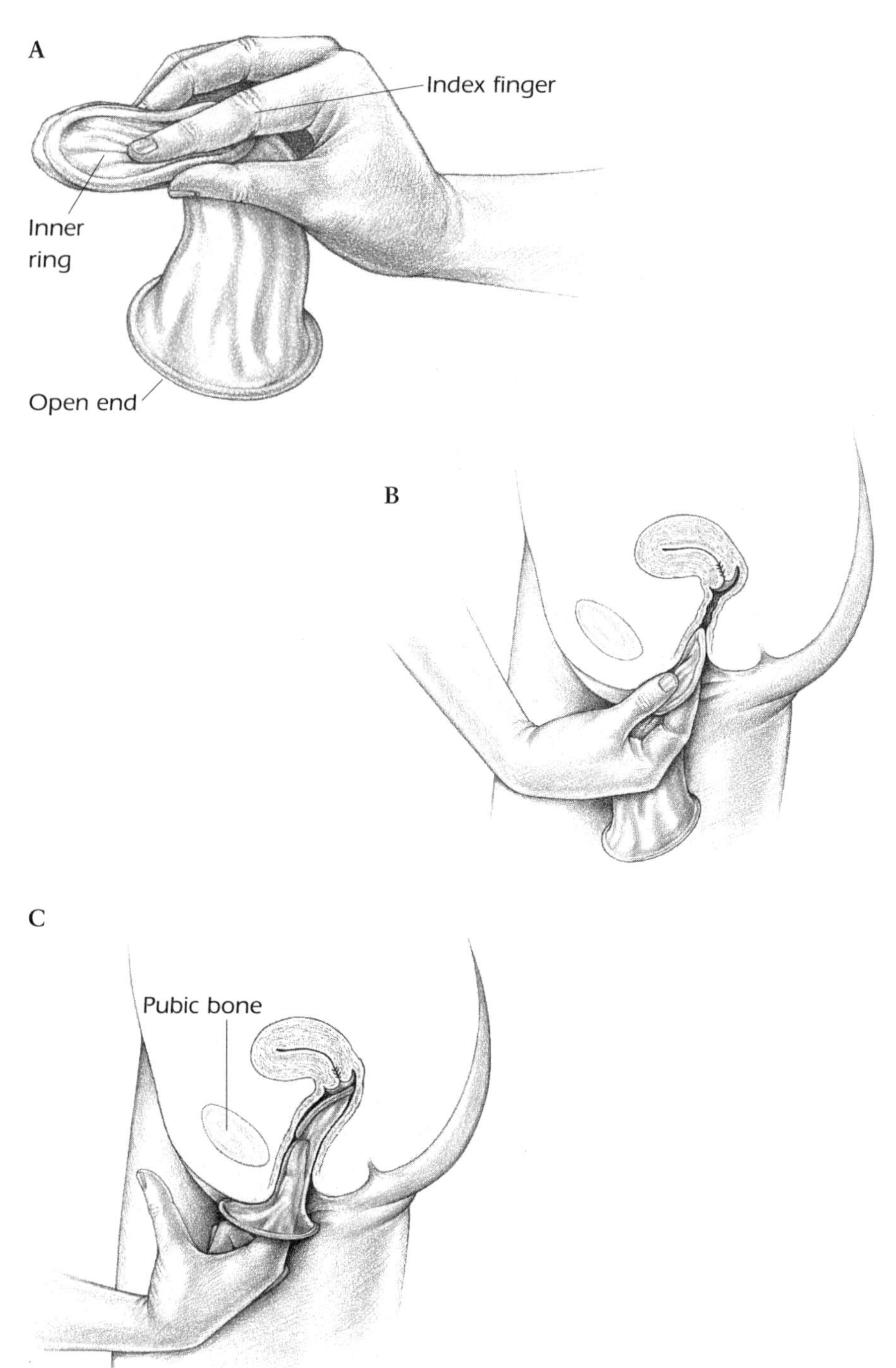

FIGURE 3.2 How to Insert a Female Condom

enough to go into your vagina. It may be easier if you squeeze it between your thumb and middle finger, with your index finger on top of the ring to help hold it steady. Be careful not to tear the condom with your fingernails or rings.

• Use your other hand to spread the outer and inner lips of your vagina and then insert the squeezed inner ring. If it slips from your fingers, let it go and start over. The condom is well lubricated, which can make it a little difficult to manage. If your vagina feels a little dry, however, you may need to add some more lubricant to the condom or to the entrance of your vagina.

• Push the inner ring and the pouch all the way up into your vagina as far as it will go. (Vaginas are about 2 1/2 to 4 inches long.) The easiest guide for doing this is to follow the lower or back wall of the vagina with the folded ring until it stops. This will help the leading edge of the ring to go under and past the cervix and touch the back wall of your vagina where it joins the cervix. The end of the folded ring closest to the vaginal opening should then be just past your pubic bone. You can feel your pubic bone—it is barely a finger's length inside the vagina. Push the ring up behind the pubic bone, which will help hold it in place. (See Chapter 1 for more information about your anatomy.)

• When the condom is in place, it covers your cervix and you should be able to feel the cervix through it. If the condom is not comfortable, it may not be correctly positioned. Remove it (twist the outer ring and gently pull) and try again. It takes a little practice to get it in place behind the pubic bone and over the cervix. Aim the leading edge a little lower so it does not hit the cervix instead of the back wall of the vagina. When you think you have the condom in place, you can check it with your finger to make sure it is over the cervix.

• About 1 inch of the open end of the condom will remain outside your vagina. While this may look unusual, it is this extra material that protects your genital area and the upper part of your partner's penis.

• Use a fresh condom for each intercourse, because the used one may have been torn or contaminated with body fluids. Do not use a

Reality and a male condom at the same time. They will stick to each other and will not stay in place.

• When you are ready to have sex, make sure the outside ring is lying flat against the outer lips of your vagina. As the penis begins to enter, guide it into the ring. If this entry is not easy, ask your partner to withdraw for a second while you add more lubricant either to his penis or to the inside of the condom. If you do not have Reality lubricant, you can use any gel or oil—polyurethane condoms are not damaged by oils.

• It is normal for the female condom to move around during sex and for the outer ring to move from side to side. It is even okay if it rides up on the penis—this does not reduce your protection because the penis is still covered and the semen stays inside the pouch.

• If you begin to feel the outer ring being pushed into the vagina or if the penis starts to enter underneath or next to the condom instead of into it, stop. You or your partner may need to add extra lubrication to the opening of the pouch and make sure the outer ring is lying flat over the lips of the vagina—this will make it easier for the penis to slide into the condom. The Reality should not bunch up if there is enough lubricant in it. It helps if you make sure the outer ring is lying flat while you guide the penis into it.

Removing the Female Condom

To remove the Reality after sex (before you stand up), squeeze the outer ring and twist it to keep any sperm from spilling. Pull gently to remove the condom, wrap it in tissues, and drop it in a trash can. Do not flush it down the toilet and do not reuse it.

COST

The only female condom on the market today is the Reality. Costs range from $7.00 to $8.99 for a package of three, and a package of six is $13.00 or more. Large drugstore chains tend to have the lowest prices.

4

The Diaphragm

The diaphragm is a shallow rubber cap with a rim made of a fine, flexible spring (Figure 4.1). It fits snugly and comfortably across the upper vagina, covering the entire cervix, thus preventing sperm from getting into the uterus and fallopian tubes to fertilize an egg. It is used with a spermicidal (sperm-killing) jelly or gel.

The diaphragm is a popular method of birth control because it does not cause any hormonal or chemical changes in the body. It has almost no side effects and does not have to interrupt lovemaking. Few men are bothered by the presence of a diaphragm, if they even notice it. It can be used during menstruation.

When used consistently and carefully, a diaphragm plus spermicide offers quite good protection against pregnancy and those sexu-

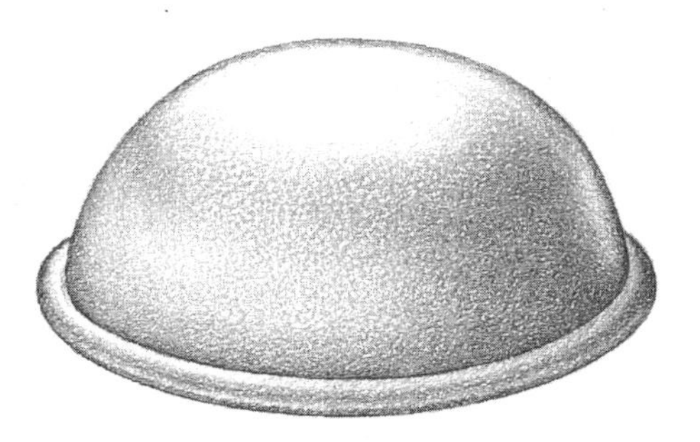

FIGURE 4.1 Diaphragm

IN A NUTSHELL

THE DIAPHRAGM

The diaphragm is a method of birth control used by a woman. It looks like a rubber cap with a flexible rim. It is always used with a spermicide (sperm-killing) gel. It is designed to fit over the cervix (at the upper end of the vagina) to prevent sperm from getting into it. You put it in place before you have sex. It prevents pregnancy and protects against some STDs, but not all. It has not been shown to protect against AIDS.

Because diaphragms must fit well to be effective, they come in several sizes. A diaphragm should fit so it stays in place but you do not feel it. A nurse or doctor must examine you and write a prescription for the correct size. With the prescription, you can buy a diaphragm at a pharmacy or a clinic. You do not need a prescription for a spermicide, which you can buy at the clinic, pharmacy, or supermarket.

You can put in the diaphragm up to 6 hours before you have sex and you must leave it in for at least 6 hours afterward.

ally transmitted diseases caused by bacteria. The risk of pelvic inflammatory disease (PID) is reduced substantially by the use of a diaphragm. Whether it protects against AIDS and other virus-caused diseases has not yet been proved.

A diaphragm needs to be fitted by a doctor or other health care provider and generally can be used for several years or longer.

The diaphragm is a particularly good method if you do not have sex frequently or if you know in advance when you will have intercourse. If you own a diaphragm but are now on the Pill, the diaphragm can provide good emergency protection if you run out of pills or are vulnerable to pregnancy because you forgot to take two or more pills. Some couples like the idea of using a contraceptive only when they believe that the woman is fertile, and they use a diaphragm, cervical cap, or condom during that time.

To be most effective, the diaphragm is used with a spermicide. It must be inserted before intercourse and must remain in place for 6 hours afterward. It should be kept handy even when you do not expect to have sex. You also need to keep a supply of spermicide on hand.

ARE YOU A GOOD CANDIDATE FOR A DIAPHRAGM?

If touching your genitals is distasteful to you, you may prefer another method of birth control.

If spontaneous, uninterrupted sex is important to you or your partner, and stopping at any point to insert the diaphragm is a nuisance that would discourage your use of it, you may want to consider another method of birth control. (To overcome this drawback, however, you can wear the diaphragm every time you are with your partner, or put it in when you get ready for bed.)

Using this contraceptive effectively also requires a certain amount of planning ahead so that you have both the diaphragm and a supply of spermicide handy. To protect it from damage, the diaphragm should be carried in its case, which is roughly 5 × 8 inches and fits into a large purse. The case often has room for a tube of spermicide. To be safe, you need to take it with you whenever you might need it. If this is not easy, another method may be a better choice.

On the other hand, the diaphragm is a good method of birth control for the woman who should not use hormonal methods because of health reasons—such as a heart problem or smoking habit.

It has a few disadvantages. If you often try different positions when having sex, you may find that the diaphragm can be dislodged when the woman is on top. This does not happen often or to everyone, but it is possible. It may depend on the woman's anatomy or the fit of the device.

During oral sex, some spermicides can leave an unpleasant taste, although this can be eliminated by wiping off your genital area after you insert the diaphragm. Both flavored and unflavored spermicidal products are available.

A spermicide is recommended because the diaphragm itself may not be completely effective in stopping sperm from entering the cervix. During intercourse, the vagina can flex and change in shape. As a result, a diaphragm cannot provide a perfect seal, and some sperm may slip past it. To protect against this possibility, a spermicidal jelly or cream is used with the diaphragm each time. One of the diaphragm's functions is to hold spermicide close to the cervical opening to destroy any sperm that get past the rim. Approximately two teaspoons of a spermicide are put in the cup of the diaphragm before it is inserted. (For more information on spermicides, see Chapter 6.)

EFFECTIVENESS

Like condoms and cervical caps, the diaphragm's effectiveness depends directly on how carefully and consistently it is used. Rates of failure vary widely, ranging from 5 to 21 percent during the first 12 months of use. Women who do not use the diaphragm every single time they have sex have the highest failure rate. Women who use it carefully every time they have sex experience the lowest rate of failure. Leaving the diaphragm at home is one of the most common reasons for failure.

Age and frequency of intercourse also affect the chance of failure. Diaphragm users who are under age 25 or who have sex frequently run a greater risk of becoming pregnant. Men and women in their teens and twenties are usually extremely fertile, which increases their risk of pregnancy. And, when intercourse is frequent, there are more chances for contraceptive failure, unless the couple is very disciplined about using this or any barrier method.

To prevent pregnancy and disease, it is necessary to use the diaphragm *every time* you have sex, even during menstruation and the so-called "safe" days shortly before or after menstruation. For greatest protection, a condom can be used in addition during the woman's most fertile days. (For information on determining your fertile and nonfertile days, see Chapter 14.)

HEALTH EFFECTS

As a rule, the diaphragm produces no serious, negative effects on the body, nor can it be lost in the vagina or in the upper reproductive tract.

Beneficial Effects

A diaphragm used with a spermicide is an effective barrier against the organisms that cause such STDs as gonorrhea, trichomoniasis, and chlamydia. In addition, cancer of the cervix has been found to be much less common in women who consistently used a diaphragm during intercourse for at least 5 years.

Urinary Tract Infections

Some women who wear diaphragms have a slightly increased risk of repeated urinary tract infections. The pressure of the rim on the urethra and bladder may be a factor in this. A diaphragm in a smaller size or with a different type of rim may exert less pressure and eliminate this possibility. As a precaution against infection, the diaphragm should be washed thoroughly with soap and water after each use, and the user should wash her hands before taking it from the case.

Toxic Shock Syndrome

Symptoms of this rare syndrome include fever, diarrhea, vomiting, muscle aches, and a sunburn-like rash, particularly on the palms of your hands and the soles of your feet. If these should occur, call your doctor. Although toxic shock is unusual, it is so serious the possibility should not be overlooked.

Allergic Reactions

In some instances, a diaphragm user or her partner is allergic to the latex or the spermicide. Women experience this problem more often than men, developing an irritation in the vagina. The cause may be a sensitivity to the perfumes used in certain brands of spermicides or to nonoxynol-9, the active ingredient. Using an unscented spermicide, or one that contains less nonoxynol-9, may solve the problem. To discover if the allergy is from the spermicide, insert some by itself into the vagina without the diaphragm. Either have no sex during this time or do this during the nonfertile days of your cycle. If you can do this for several days without irritation, the spermicide is probably not the cause.

Instead of an allergy, sometimes vaginal soreness is just the result of irritation from the spermicide. Talk to your health care provider about this problem and about using another, nonirritating form of contraception. Condoms may provide a solution, and the cervical cap is another choice. Since it requires very little spermicide, the cap can sometimes be a good method for women who tend to be irritated by spermicides (see Chapter 5).

If the spermicide is not the source of the irritation, latex is the likely suspect. Since all diaphragms today are made of latex, if you want to continue with a barrier method, the only nonlatex choices are the new polyurethane or Tactylon male condoms (Chapter 2) or the female condom (Chapter 3).

USING THE DIAPHRAGM

Diaphragms are available from women's health centers and Planned Parenthood clinics, from physicians, particularly family practitioners and gynecologists, and from nurse-midwives, nurse-practitioners, and other health professionals specializing in family planning. Spermicides are also available from these sources or from the feminine hygiene or family planning sections in drugstores.

Types of Diaphragms

Diaphragms are available in sizes measured in millimeters, ranging from 50 to 95 millimeters (about 2 to 4 inches) in diameter. The size you need depends on the size of your upper vagina, which is related to your body size and weight, as well as whether you experienced a vaginal childbirth. Diaphragms are available with different types of rims that make it possible to fit many different bodies.

The diaphragm with a *flat spring rim* exerts a very gentle pressure. It is often the best choice for the woman whose vaginal muscles are very firm because she has not yet had a baby. A *coil spring rim* is stronger and is designed for the vagina with a more relaxed muscle wall. A diaphragm with an *arcing spring rim* bends in only two places, which some women find easier to handle.

Both the arcing spring and coil spring types are available with an extra "wide seal" inner rim of soft latex. This is intended to create a better seal with the vaginal wall and to be more effective in holding the spermicide around the cervix.

Being Fitted

Because the diaphragm must fit very well, it is necessary to have an internal pelvic examination by a physician or other health care provider. The examination rules out any problem that would prevent you from using a diaphragm successfully, such as an abnormality of the vagina, cervix, or uterus. This is also a good time to ask to be examined for infections of the lower reproductive tract. Many infections have no symptoms and without a lab test they could remain undiscovered. They should be treated before they cause complications.

If you are under age 18 and wonder if the clinic or physician will tell your parents about your visit, you may find it helpful to ask some of the privacy questions listed on page 234 in Chapter 18.

During the exam, the practitioner will assess which type and size of diaphragm will suit your body best. This usually is done with fitting rings or sample diaphragms, and several may have to be tried to find the size that is comfortable and secure in the vagina. The ideal is the largest model that is snug without discomfort. A diaphragm is a good fit if it touches the walls of the vagina with just enough room to insert a fingertip beneath the pubic bone.

If you are not at ease with the idea of inserting and removing a diaphragm by hand, some types can be used with a plastic inserter. Discuss this possibility with your practitioner.

Part of the fitting procedure must include a lesson on how to insert and remove the diaphragm. You should be given plenty of opportunity to practice while you are still in the examining room. If the rim is too stiff to be squeezed together by one hand, a model with a less firm spring may be preferable. Although more practice with the diaphragm will make it easier to use, you should feel fairly confident about inserting it before you leave the clinic.

If you wish, it usually is possible to take the diaphragm home to practice inserting it and then, while wearing it, go back to your practitioner to make sure it is in the right place. This is not possible if you are simply given a prescription for buying the diaphragm at a drugstore.

You want to be able to put it in and take it out correctly and easily before you actually use the diaphragm. If it is a good fit, you should not be able to feel it. It may be too large if you feel the need to urinate shortly after you put it in or if you have a sense of pressure on your abdomen. When abdominal pain or cramping or vaginal pressure accompany the presence of the diaphragm, its position and size should be checked. Do not accept one that causes you any discomfort when it is correctly placed.

How to Insert the Diaphragm

- Before putting in the diaphragm, wash your hands. If you are not familiar with the anatomy of your vagina and cervix, you will find it easier to use this method if you know where your cervix and pubic bone are (see Chapter 1) and what they feel like. There is no need to be embarrassed—after all, this is an important part of your body and you should know about it.
- Fill the diaphragm almost two-thirds full of a spermicide (a couple of inches or about 2 or 3 teaspoons). How much you need depends on its size: a larger one will require more spermicide. Spread it around and up on the inside of the rim. For extra protection, some women smear a bit of spermicide on the outside of the diaphragm or put a dab on one spot of the outer rim, which is less messy. Avoid making the outside of the rim too slippery—you may find the diaphragm flying out of your hand!
- You can insert the diaphragm while sitting on the toilet, or lying down with your legs bent, or in a squatting position—whatever works for you (Figure 4.2). If you sit on the toilet, take care that the rim of the diaphragm is not slippery from spermicide because it may slip from your hands.

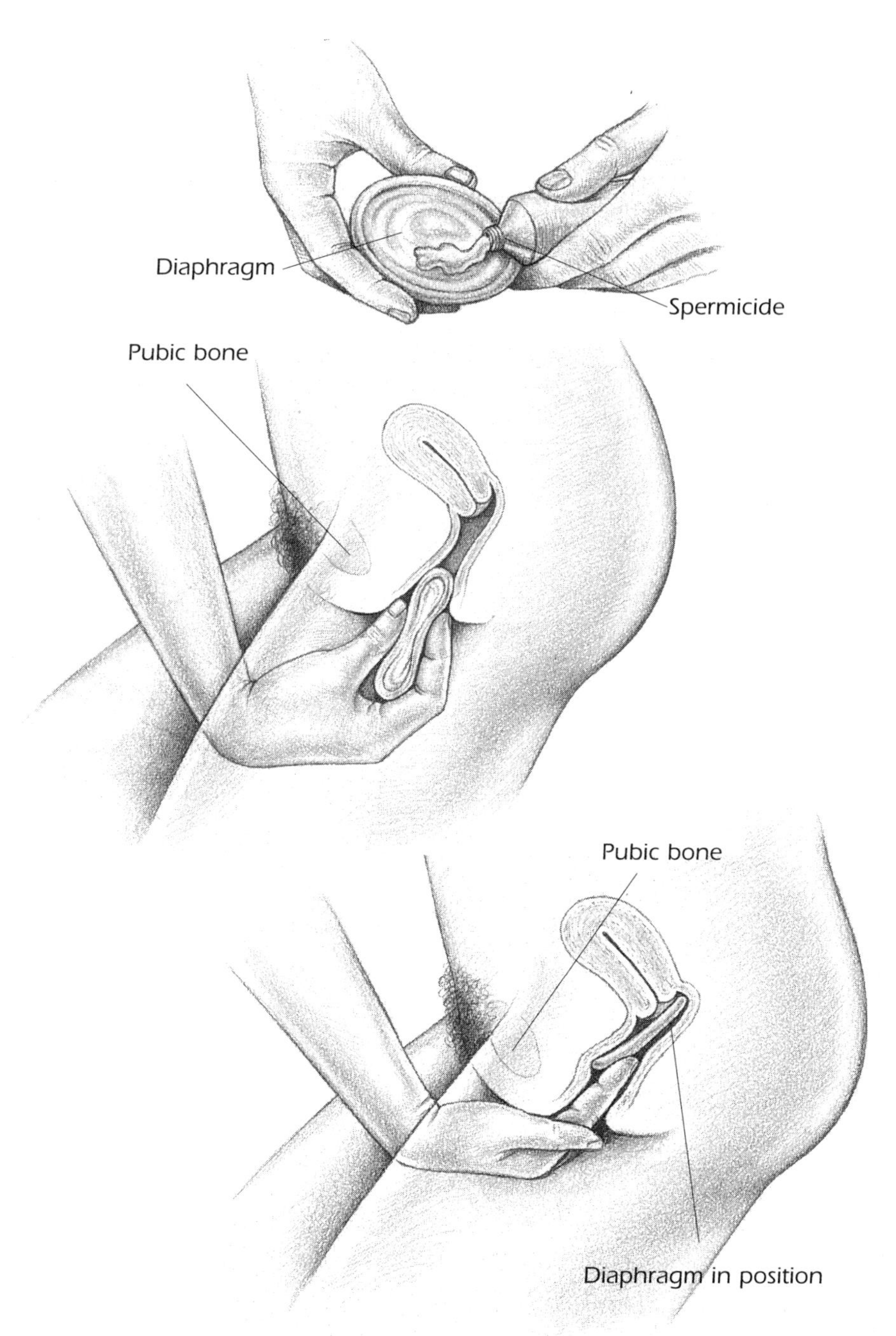

FIGURE 4.2 How to Insert a Diaphragm

• If you ever drop your diaphragm, wash it well with soap and water, add spermicide, and start over.

• With the open side of the cup facing upward, firmly squeeze the sides of the rim together between your thumb and fingers to fold it for insertion. If the spermicide has made the rim too slippery to grasp, wipe it from the outer edge only, not from the inside. A little spermicide in one spot on the leading edge, however, does help it slide more easily into the vagina.

• While you hold the folded diaphragm in one hand, spread apart the lips of the vagina with the other hand and then ease the diaphragm up into the vaginal canal as far back as it will go—about two or three inches. The leading edge of the rim should slip under and behind the cervix and touch the vaginal wall. Then gently but firmly push the other edge up behind the pubic bone. When it is in the correct position, the diaphragm should cover the cervix, feel comfortable, and stay in place.

• Use your longest finger to make sure the rim of the diaphragm closest to the vaginal opening is tucked up behind the pubic bone and that the cervix is covered by the soft rubber dome. Your cervix is at the upper end of your vagina—it feels like the tip of your nose—and you should be able to feel it through the latex. Touching it through the diaphragm also makes sure the spermicide is in contact with the cervical opening, protecting it from sperm.

• If you are aware of your diaphragm when you are wearing it, it is probably not correctly placed. Take it out and try again. Try sitting differently when you insert it. Also make more of an effort to keep the leading edge of the diaphragm low so it goes under the cervix. Remember that using any barrier method is awkward at first and it takes a little practice before the diaphragm becomes easy to insert.

The Spermicide

Spermicides lose their effectiveness in the body as time passes. If you inserted the diaphragm more than two hours before actually having sex, squeeze another application directly into your vagina.

NOTE: Do not take out the diaphragm when you add more spermicide.

To use the plastic applicator that comes with the spermicide, remove the cap from the tube and attach the applicator in its place. Squeeze the tube so the jelly, gel, or cream pushes into the applicator and fills it. Disconnect the applicator and insert it well into your vagina, just as you would a tampon, and then gently push the plunger in as far as it will go. When you remove the applicator, do not tug on the plunger because that might pull some of the cream back into it. Contraceptive foams, available in most drugstores, can be used with diaphragms instead of a cream or gel (for more information on spermicide products, see Chapter 6). You can apply the spermicide in the bathroom or while still in bed. It takes only a moment.

As we noted in the chapter on condoms (Chapter 2), when you use a latex device, it is vital not to use petroleum jelly or any other oil-based ointment or cream instead of a spermicide. For one thing, these products do not kill sperm. For another, any product with oil in it weakens latex and causes it to develop tiny holes that allow sperm, viruses, and bacteria to pass through. If you want to use a lubricant during intercourse, use your spermicide or a water-based vaginal lubricant such as K-Y Jelly, Ortho-Gynol, or Koromex Gel. When you buy a lubricant, read the label carefully to make sure it is safe to use with latex.

Afterward

After sex is over, leave the diaphragm in place for at least 6 hours. It takes that long for the spermicide to kill all the sperm. Although in some cases the diaphragm can be dislodged if the vagina flexes a great deal during intercourse, you can safely take a bath, shower, swim, bicycle, and perform almost any kind of physical activity without it moving out of place. You also can have a bowel movement without dislodging it. Do not douche while wearing a diaphragm. Douching washes away protective spermicides and can force sperm up the cervix.

You can leave the diaphragm in place for longer than 8 hours, and many women prefer to do so. In fact, it is usually more convenient to wait until morning to remove it. But do not leave it in for more than 24 hours at a stretch. Leaving barriers in place for extended periods of time may be associated with increased risk of toxic shock syndrome.

Further Intercourse

Before having more sex, add an applicator of spermicide. If 8 or more hours have passed, and you expect to have intercourse again, you can remove and wash the diaphragm if you wish, add more spermicide, and reinsert it. Or you can just leave the diaphragm in place and add more spermicide.

Removing the Diaphragm

Before removing the diaphragm, again, wash your hands. Then find a comfortable position. Hook a finger under the part of the diaphragm that rests behind the pubic bone or at any other point

DIAPHRAGM POINTERS

- Do not forget to take your diaphragm with you when you go on vacation or away for the weekend. If you travel frequently, keep a second diaphragm and supply of spermicide in your travel kit.
- Always keep a tube of spermicide and applicator with your diaphragm in its case.
- If your diaphragm becomes dislodged during intercourse, immediately add more spermicide well into the vagina. Talk to your health care provider as soon as possible about emergency contraception (see Chapter 16).
- If you are not sure that you are inserting the diaphragm correctly, or if it does not feel comfortable, have the placement checked by the health care provider who fitted you. Meanwhile, have your partner use a condom for extra protection. (It is always a good idea to keep a supply of condoms on hand.)

toward the front of the vagina. Firmly pull forward and down. If it is a good fit, it may take a bit of effort to dislodge the diaphragm. Be careful not to poke a fingernail through it. Because a certain amount of sperm and contraceptive cream will come out of the vagina with the diaphragm, many women remove their diaphragms while sitting on the toilet. The use of a minipad or tampon will protect you against any leakage afterward.

CARE AND STORAGE

Simple care extends a diaphragm's life and effectiveness. After using it, wash it with soap and warm water, rinse, and pat it dry with a clean towel. (A diaphragm should not be put away while still wet.) Do not use antiseptics or strong cleansing solutions on a diaphragm, because they weaken the latex. To protect it further, before returning it to its case, dust the diaphragm with cornstarch—not talcum or any other perfumed powders; the perfumes can damage it. Store your diaphragm in its case and do not expose it to sunlight or extreme heat.

Examine your diaphragm every few weeks for holes, especially around the rim. Even the tiniest pinhole can admit hundreds of sperm. To make a check, hold it up to the light and look at it carefully. Or fill it with water to see if it leaks. The latex will gradually grow darker with time; this is all right, it does not affect its function. Replace the diaphragm when the rubber shows signs of deterioration, such as cracks or brittleness.

CHECKING YOUR DIAPHRAGM

Your diaphragm and its fit should be checked every 18 months or so. This can be done when you have your regular pelvic exam and Pap smear. The fit should also be checked in the following circumstances:

- if you have lost or gained more than 20 pounds;
- if you have had a child, a miscarriage, an abortion, or any type of surgery involving your reproductive organs;

- anytime you experience discomfort, pain, or recurring bladder infections after using the diaphragm; or
- anytime you suspect your diaphragm is not fitting properly or that you might not be inserting it correctly.

COST

The medical examination and a diaphragm fitting can cost from $75 to $150 or more, depending on where you live and who does it. Women's health centers, state or city family planning clinics, and Planned Parenthood clinics usually offer the lowest costs. The most expensive source may be your gynecologist. However, if you have been having regular pelvic examinations, your gynecologist, internist, family practitioner, or adolescent medicine specialist may do just the fitting procedure for less than the cost of an exam. The cost of the diaphragm may be included.

Prices of spermicidal gels, jellies, and creams begin at $8 and the tubes vary in the number of ounces they hold. An ounce of spermicide is equal to 6 teaspoons or 2 to 3 applications. A 3.8 ounce tube contains about 10 applications. Read the label to be sure the contents actually are a spermicidal—are intended to kill sperm. Some vaginal lubricants that do not contain nonoxynol-9 (the active sperm-killing ingredient) are sold in similar packages, although they usually are much cheaper. Contraceptive foams and gels often are available at reduced cost from Planned Parenthood and other family planning clinics.

If you need to replace your diaphragm, it is usually not necessary to have another pelvic examination. If you make a note of the size of your diaphragm, the health care practitioner who provided it can telephone a prescription for a new one to your pharmacy. The size is usually printed on the rim. It should also be noted in your medical records.

5

The Cervical Cap

The cervical cap is a small, deep latex cup with a firm but flexible rim around the open end. It is 1 1/4 to 1 1/2 inches long and looks like a large rubber thimble. It fits snugly over the cervix and the *os*, the tiny opening to the cervix (Figure 5.1).

The cervical cap is similar to a diaphragm in that it does not cause any hormonal or chemical changes in the body. It has almost no side effects and does not interrupt lovemaking. When used for every single act of intercourse, the cap plus spermicide offers very good protection against pregnancy and some sexually transmitted

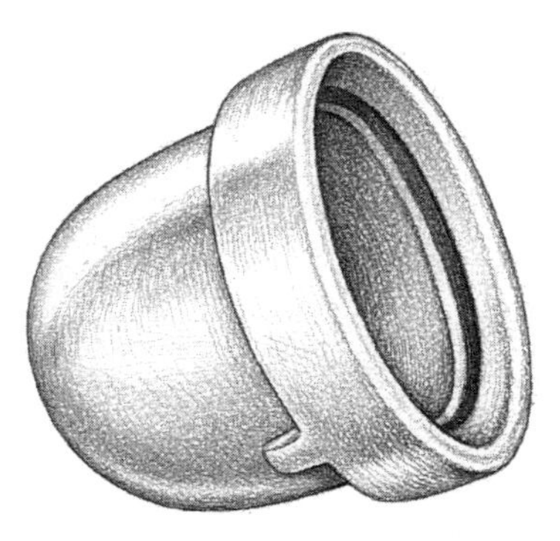

FIGURE 5.1 The Prentif Cervical Cap

IN A NUTSHELL

THE CERVICAL CAP

The cervical cap is a small, deep rubber cap that fits tightly over the cervix to prevent sperm from entering. It is used with a spermicide. You push the cap up your vagina and over the cervix anytime before you have sex. It must be left in place for at least 6 hours afterward, but you can wear it for as long as 48 hours.

A cervical cap protects you against pregnancy and some STDs. It does not protect against AIDS and the other STDs that are caused by viruses.

Cervical caps come in four sizes. Your clinic nurse or doctor will examine you to see if you can use the cap. With a prescription for the correct size you can buy a cap from the clinic. You also can buy the spermicide you will need at a pharmacy or the clinic.

diseases. It has not been shown to protect against AIDS and other virus-caused STDs.

Although the cervical cap functions like a diaphragm, it has a different shape, fits differently, and is used with less spermicide. It is held in place by suction, by its close fit on the cervix, and by the slight pressure of the surrounding vaginal wall.

Like the diaphragm, a cap requires a physical examination, including a Pap smear, and a fitting session. The standard fitting procedure also includes a follow-up Pap smear after the cap has been used for 3 months. A cervical cap usually needs to be replaced every 12 to 18 months.

A cervical cap has an advantage over the diaphragm because you can insert the cap many hours before having sex and, afterward, you can leave it in place longer.

The main disadvantage is that the only type of cervical cap available in the United States at this time (the Prentif cap) is made in just four sizes. Because anatomy varies, about 20 percent of women cannot get a good fit with the Prentif.

If you often try different positions while having intercourse, you may find that in some positions the cervical cap can be dislodged. This depends largely on the anatomy of your cervix, the fit of the cap, and the respective sizes of the vagina and penis.

The cervical cap has been used in Europe since the 19th century, but it was not approved for general use in the United States until 1988. It is still not well known here, and many physicians are not familiar with this method. Women's health centers and some health maintenance organizations are more likely to have the cap available.

EFFECTIVENESS

In studies of the effectiveness of the cap in preventing pregnancy, failure rates ranged from 8 to 19 percent—or 8 to 19 pregnancies per 100 women during the first year of use. It also is considered a good, but not perfect, method of protection against STDs. Because it covers the cervix, it protects the upper reproductive tract against sperm and bacteria. However, it does not protect the vagina against bacteria, and whether it prevents virus-caused diseases, such as AIDS, is not proven.

As with other barrier contraceptives, the effectiveness of this method depends largely on how faithfully it is used. To protect yourself against pregnancy and disease, you must wear a cervical cap every time you have sex.

The cap cannot be used during menstruation because it does not permit any flow of secretions from the cervix. A male or female condom or a diaphragm are good birth control methods if you have intercourse during menstruation.

A disadvantage of the cap is that it can become dislodged during sex if it hasn't been put on correctly in the first place or if it does not fit securely because of the shape of the cervix. You can sometimes avoid having it come off by using a different position during intercourse. An experienced cap fitter may be able to tell you, based on your anatomy, what positions to avoid and what might be preferable.

You can improve the effectiveness of the cervical cap by adding a backup method during the first months you use the cap. Use a backup until you know from experience that you are placing the cap properly and it will not be dislodged. Another approach is to avoid intercourse or use condoms or extra spermicide during the most fertile days of your cycle. (For information on fertile days, see Chapter 14.)

NOT EVERY WOMAN CAN WEAR A CERVICAL CAP

The Prentif is the only cap available in the United States and not all women can wear it. Prentif caps come in four sizes and do not fit all women, largely because of ordinary variations in the anatomy of the individual cervix.

If the cervix has uneven sides, is exceptionally long or short, or is irregularly shaped, it usually is impossible to achieve the snug fit necessary for effective birth control. If the uterus is extremely anteflexed—bent so the cervix points back toward the spine–the cap could easily be dislodged.

A woman may not be able to use a cervical cap because she has a very long vagina and cannot reach her cervix to place a cap on it. An experienced cervical cap fitter can usually identify these problems.

HEALTH EFFECTS

The cervical cap seldom has negative health effects. There is a theoretical risk of toxic shock syndrome if you wear the cap for more than 72 hours, although no documented cases exist. To avoid the possibility of toxic shock, do not wear the cap for more than 48 hours or during menstruation. As we noted in Chapter 4, the symptoms of toxic shock syndrome include fever, muscle aches, diarrhea, and vomiting. The most distinctive symptom, however, is a sunburn-like rash on the palms of the hands and the soles of your feet. If you ever have had toxic shock you should not use the cervical cap.

If you suspect toxic shock, remove the cap immediately and, as soon as possible, call your doctor. If fewer than 6 hours have passed since you have had sex, insert an applicator of spermicide before you remove the cap.

If you ever have to remove the cap before 6 hours have elapsed, especially during your fertile period, you may want to discuss emergency contraception with your physician or family planning clinic. (See Chapter 16 for more information on emergency contraception.)

Unlike the diaphragm, the cervical cap exerts no pressure on the urinary tract, and it is seldom associated with an increase in urinary tract infections.

Cervical Changes

In a study of cervical cap use sponsored by the National Institutes of Health, 4 percent of the women who entered the study with normal Pap tests developed cervical tissue abnormalities during their first 3 months of using the cap. Researchers theorize that the layer of cells that lines the cervix may become more vulnerable to the human papilloma virus when a cervical cap is used regularly. Several of the many strains of human papilloma virus are associated with, or cause, cancer of the cervix. For this reason, the FDA has recommended that a Pap test be performed before a cap is fitted and again after three months of use. If either test shows any abnormal cells, another form of contraception should be adopted.

Allergic Reactions

If a woman has developed an allergy to latex, she should not use the cap. Even without a latex allergy, there is always a slight risk that using the cap may irritate the cervix or the penis. The cause may be a sensitivity to the perfumes used in certain brands of spermicides or to nonoxynol-9, the active ingredient. To see if the irritation may be caused by the spermicide, switch to a different, unperfumed product or one with a lower percentage of nonoxynol-9 and apply it without the cap. If the irritation clears up after a number of days, use the new spermicide instead. If you think you may be allergic to latex, you should discuss this with the practitioner who fitted you with the cap. Since the latex Prentif is the only cervical cap available at this time, you may have to use another method.

Sometimes irritation is caused simply by leaving the cap on too long. The cap can be worn up to 48 hours after sex, and it must be left in place for at least 6 hours after intercourse. An irritation may subside if you use the cap for just that minimum length of time.

It is important not to tolerate a badly irritated cervix or vagina. The tiny cracks in the sore tissues may provide an opening for infection. If the irritation does not clear up in a short time, talk to your health care provider about it. In the meanwhile, your best protection is the nonlatex, polyurethane male condom sold under the name Avanti (see Chapter 2), or the polyurethane Reality female condom (see Chapter 3).

Future Options for the Allergic

A new type of cervical cap made of silicone rubber is currently being tested for its effectiveness and safety in actual use. This form of rubber does not irritate and is soft, durable, easy to clean, and can be sterilized. It also is not easily damaged by heat, body fluids, or oil-based products. Called the Femcap, it is expected to become available sometime in late 1998.

USING THE CERVICAL CAP

If you live in a large city or town, the best way to find a source of cervical caps is to check the telephone yellow pages under clinics, health services, or women's health services. Although a woman's health center is more likely than a physician to be able to fit a cervical cap, you certainly should tell your gynecologist if you are interested in this form of birth control. Some health maintenance organizations (HMOs) also are now offering this method.

If you are under age 18 and wonder if the clinic or physician will tell your parents about your visit, you may find it helpful to ask some of the privacy questions listed on page 234 in Chapter 18.

Being Fitted

The Prentif is a deep cap, almost 1 1/2 inches long. It is made of latex with a sturdy rim. On the inside of the rim is a groove that enhances the cap's ability to cling to the cervix. The Prentif comes in four sizes, with inside diameters of 22, 25, 28, and 31 millimeters.

Some days of the month are better than others for being fitted for a cervical cap. The best time is midcycle, between days 10 and 18. (Day 1 of the cycle is the first day of menstruation.) First, your health care provider will take your medical history, do a thorough pelvic examination, and perform a Pap test. The purpose of this is to discover any medical or anatomical problem involving the cervix, such as an irregular shape, that might make it impossible for a cap to achieve a good seal. If you have had a pelvic exam and Pap test within the preceding 3 months, you should not have to repeat this, the most expensive part of the exam, if you can get a note or a copy of the test results from the practitioner who performed the exam.

A cap cannot be fitted during menstruation, or when there is a vaginal or cervical infection. Nor can it be fitted during the weeks after childbirth or abortion or any procedure that involves the cervix, such as a dilatation and curettage (D&C). During the physical exam, the practitioner will assess whether the anatomy of your cervix makes you a good candidate for a cap and what size you are most likely to need. She will use sample caps to find the best fit.

To achieve a good fit, the inner diameter of the cap must be only a millimeter or two larger than the cervix. When the cap is in place, there should be no space between the rim and the cervix, and the cap should be deep enough that its top does not rest right on the opening of the cervix.

Because differences in anatomy affect the way the cap fits, it is a good idea to ask your practitioner just how well it covers your cervix. If the fit involves any unusual features, you want to be aware of them so you know when your cap is in the right place. For instance, if you have a long cervix, a cap might not completely cover it.

If you have any questions about cap placement or the security of its seal, or if the cap is uncomfortable, arrange for a fitting check after you have put it on at home.

How To Insert the Cap

Some women find inserting and removing the cervical cap a bit more difficult than using a diaphragm. Other women find that the cap requires less effort because it is smaller and easier to move through the vagina. With practice at home, most are able to slide it into place easily (Figure 5.2). Take all the time you need at your doctor's office or clinic until you feel sure that you are putting the cap in and taking it out with ease. In addition, sitting in on a cervical

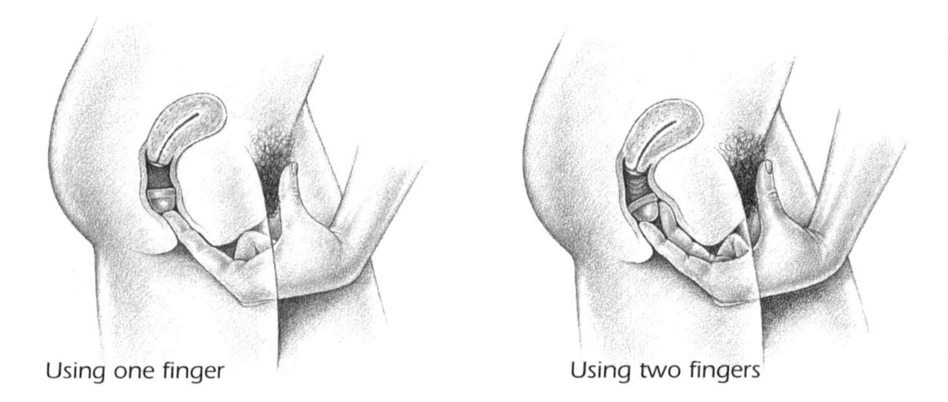

FIGURE 5.2 Placing Cap on Cervix

cap self-help group—if one is available—helps to ensure that you receive an adequate fit and are satisfied with this birth control method. Practitioners who fit caps are good sources for finding such a group.

• Before inserting the cap, locate your cervix with your fingers. Because its position changes throughout your menstrual cycle, knowing its current position makes it easier to put the cap in place.

• To make sure it is comfortable, practice inserting the cap several times and wear it for 8 hours before you actually use it for intercourse.

• To test its fit, remove the cap after 20 minutes and see if you can feel a raised ring around your cervix. If you can, your cap has a good, snug fit. If there is no ring, the cap may be too loose and you should tell your clinician.

• Before inserting your cap, empty your bladder and wash your hands. Choose a comfortable position: squatting, lying down with your legs bent, sitting on the edge of a sturdy chair, standing with one foot propped on a chair or the edge of the bathtub, or sitting on the toilet. (If you drop the cap, pick it up and wash it with soap and warm water.) Experiment until you find a position that works for you.

• Fill one-third of the dome with a spermicide. Do not use more; too much spermicide can prevent a good seal and may make it easier for the cap to come off during intercourse. Do not put spermicide into the hollow groove in the inside of the rim—it needs to be empty to hold onto the cervix—but do put a dab in one spot on the outer rim to make it easier to slide the cap into the vagina. You improve your protection if you also add an applicator of spermicide to your vagina after you insert the cap.

• Like the condom and the diaphragm, the cervical cap is latex and so can be damaged by any oil-based substance. If you want to use a lubricant during sex, try K-Y Jelly, H-R Lubricating Jelly, Surgilube, or any other water-based product available in drugstores.

• Pinch the edges of the cap together between your thumb and first finger. With your other hand spread apart the vaginal lips. Push the cap gently up into the vagina and along its back wall, with the opening facing up and the dome down. When your thumb can no longer reach far enough, use one or two of your longest fingers to move the cap along to the cervix. Push the cap on over the end of the cervix. Although this can be done with one finger, it is easier if you place the index finger on one side of the cap and the middle finger on the other and push it on. Then use those fingers to press around the entire rim to make certain the cap is pushed on as far as it will go and is securely in place.

• If it is hard for you to reach your cervix on certain days, try a squatting position or else bear down with your abdominal muscles as if you were having a bowel movement. This pressure pushes your cervix lower into the vagina. As we mentioned earlier, the cervix moves higher and lower in the vagina, depending on the time of month. If you continue to have difficulty inserting the cap, remove it, wait until you are more relaxed, and try again. You may want to try another position and check where your cervix is again.

Checking the Placement

When the cap is in place, use your longest finger to make sure the cap is positioned completely over the cervix (Figure 5.3). Experi-

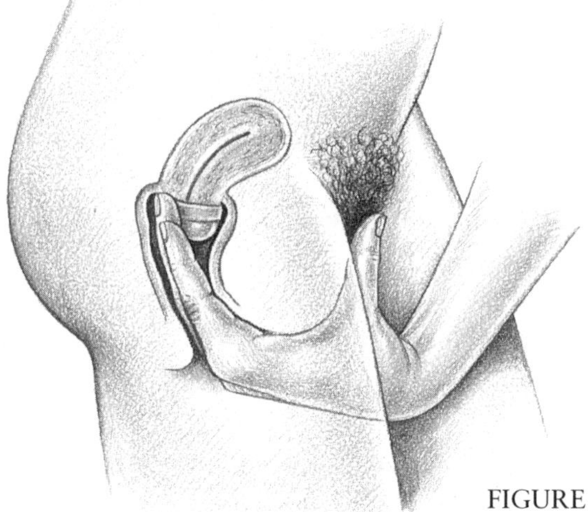

FIGURE 5.3 Checking Cap Placement

enced fitters recommend checking at the back of the cap, where the cervix is easier to feel and recognize. If the cap is on properly, it should completely cover the cervix, including its sides—to where they meet the vaginal walls. The cap should not really touch the tip of the cervix. Its top or dome should not feel tight but should "dimple in" when you touch it. You should not be able to knock the cap loose. A well-fitting cap is difficult to remove.

If the cap is not correctly positioned, either straighten it with your fingers or remove it and reinsert it. Checking its position on the cervix is important because a cap can stick to the vaginal wall instead of sliding up to and on the cervix.

Positioning the cap sounds much more difficult and complex than it actually is. All barrier contraceptives take some practice at the beginning but using them soon becomes quick and almost automatic.

Insert the cap at least 20 to 30 minutes before sex so that a good seal can develop. If you have been wearing the cap for several hours before you have intercourse, make sure it is securely in place before you begin lovemaking. You can do this in the bathroom or in bed.

CERVICAL CAP POINTERS

For the first few weeks or months that you use the cap—until you have enough experience with it to feel certain you are using it correctly and know it will not be dislodged—back it up with extra spermicide or a male condom. If the cap does become loose during sex, try different positions to find one that does not dislodge it. Use a backup contraceptive method while you are experimenting. If the cap still comes loose, return to your health care provider to try to resolve the problem.

It is not a good idea to wear the cap during those days of your period when blood flow is heavy. If blood spills over the rim, it breaks the seal between the cap and the cervix. Since it is sometimes possible to become pregnant during menstruation, you or your partner should use another form of birth control at this time.

If the Cap Becomes Dislodged

Displacement of the cap occurs most often when the penis is able to reach the cervix. The angle of the cervix or the angle of penetration may cause the penis to bump the side of the cap rather than its top, pushing it out of place. Soon after intercourse, check to see whether the cap is still firmly on the cervix. If it is loose, push it back on and immediately add an applicator of spermicide well back into the vagina. If it is completely dislodged, remove it, put some spermicide in the cap if necessary, and replace it. Then add the extra spermicide. If the cap becomes dislodged frequently, even when you use a different position for sex, see the health care provider who fitted you. You may have to consider using another birth control method.

If the cap is dislodged during intercourse, you may want to discuss emergency contraception with your health care provider. To be most effective, emergency contraception should be started within 72 hours after intercourse (see Chapter 16).

The Spermicide

To put spermicide into the vagina, remove the top of the tube and attach the applicator in its place. (Applicators are included in "starter" packages of spermicide.) Squeeze the tube until the applicator is full, disconnect it, and insert the applicator up into your vaginal canal, much like a tampon. Gently push the plunger as far as it can go. Remove the applicator without tugging on the plunger, which could pull up some of the spermicide.

If you have intercourse later while the cap is still in place, leave it on. You may add more spermicide to your vagina if you wish.

Afterward

After intercourse, leave the cap in place for at least 6 hours. If it is convenient, you can leave it in for as long as a day or two. Most practitioners recommend that the cap not be worn more than 2 days at a time, largely because of the odor caused by exposing it to vaginal secretions. In addition, not enough is known about the long-term effects of blocking the flow of normal cervical secretions and the risk of toxic shock syndrome. However, some women can wear a cap almost constantly without a problem. They remove it every other day or once a day for a few hours to wash it and to allow cervical secretions to flow freely.

Do not douche while wearing a cervical cap, because you could dilute the spermicide or force sperm into the cap. The douching solution also might make holes in the rubber.

Removing the Cap

To remove the cap, it is necessary to break the force of the seal. After you have worn the cap for some hours, the cervix swells slightly, creating an even tighter fit. With experience you will learn how much effort you need to loosen it.

After finding a good position, hook a finger over the back rim of the cap and pull. Or push the dome forward or upward with your first finger while your middle finger hooks over the back rim and pulls down. If sometimes you cannot reach the cap, even when bearing down with your abdominal muscles, ask your practitioner for the diaphragm introducer (the Universal Introducer). It has a small hook on one end that is useful for removing cervical caps.

CARE AND STORAGE

Whenever you remove it, wash the cap with a mild, unscented soap and warm water. Turn it inside out in order to clean the hollow groove inside the rim. Use a strong flow of warm water or a soft toothbrush on the groove. Do not boil the cap or use strong cleaners.

Dry the cap and, if you are not going to use it soon, dust it lightly with cornstarch to help protect the rubber from contact with anything greasy. *Do not use talcum or baby powders,* because they can cause rubber to deteriorate. Such scented powders also can irritate your vagina.

Do not rest your cervical cap on newspaper, because it often contains materials that can perforate rubber. Keep the cap away from extreme heat and sunlight because these, too, cause rubber to deteriorate. Store the cap in its container.

If an unpleasant odor develops when you wear your cervical cap for long periods, you may need to remove it more often, at least once a day, for cleaning. You often can neutralize odor by soaking the cap in lemon juice, mouthwash, or a mild solution of one teaspoon of white or cider vinegar to a quart of water. Soak it for 20 minutes. The vinegar solution will turn the cap brown, but this will not affect its reliability. Rinse it thoroughly in warm water and dry it. Odors also can be removed by adding a drop of liquid chlorophyll to the cap *before* using it or by soaking it in a cup of water mixed with a drop of chlorophyll. Chlorophyll is available from pharmacies and from some natural food stores. Do not soak the cap for more than 20 to 30 minutes.

If you have a vaginal infection, wash and sterilize the cap in rubbing alcohol (available from drugstores) for 15 minutes each time you remove it. It is also a good idea to have your partner wear a condom for his protection until the infection is cleared up.

The regular use of alcohol and acidic solutions such as vinegar and water or lemon juice hasten the deterioration of rubber. At the first sign of any cracking, hardness, stickiness, or an odor you cannot get rid of, get a new cap. Generally speaking, caps should be replaced every year. How long each one lasts depends on how often you use it, the effect of your body on the latex, and how well you take care of it.

Checking Your Cap

Every time you use your cap, examine it for holes, cracks, and signs of wear. Hold it up to the light or check for leaks by filling it with water. Have it checked when you have your annual pelvic exam and Pap smear. Your health care provider may observe changes in the cap you have not noticed. The rubber may be slightly deteriorating or the shape may have altered so it no longer provides a tight seal.

The fit of a cap should also be tested after childbirth, a miscarriage, or an abortion. After a birth, the cervix takes about 6 weeks to return to normal size. The fit should also be checked after any surgery on the cervix, including laser, electrocautery, or cryotherapy, and after any gynecological procedure in which the cervix is dilated, such as a D&C. If you are breastfeeding when you are fitted with your cap, have the size checked when you are once again menstruating—your cervix may have become larger. And if you were fitted while you were on oral contraceptives, have the fit tested after you have your first spontaneous period off the Pill.

WHERE TO GET THE CERVICAL CAP

States with large populations and large cities are likely to have numerous health professionals trained to fit cervical caps. In states with fewer people, the number of practitioners fitting caps is still relatively small, although it continues to grow. To find a provider near you, contact Cervical Cap Ltd., 430 Monterey Avenue, Suite 1B, Los Gatos, CA 95030, 408-395-2100, for an updated list for your area.

COST

A cervical cap, the fitting procedure, and a pelvic examination and Pap smear will range in cost from $100 to $200. If you have a choice of providers, it is wise to shop around because prices can vary even within the same city.

• 6 •

Spermicides

As the name implies, a spermicide is a chemical compound that kills sperm. Spermicides are available in a number of forms that are safe and easy to use—aerosol foams, gels or jellies that require an applicator, dissolvable suppositories, and dissolvable squares of film. The active ingredient in these products is nonoxynol-9, which works by damaging the surface membrane of the sperm cell. Like other barrier contraceptives, spermicides do not affect hormone levels in the body or change the environment of the uterus.

Spermicide products require no physical examination or prescription. They can be found in the feminine hygiene or family planning sections of drugstores, discount department stores, and some large supermarkets. They also are available from women's health centers, HMOs, and family planning clinics.

A spermicide can be inserted ahead of time without the need for a partner's involvement, and its presence seldom can be distinguished from the natural lubrication of the vagina. Furthermore, some types of spermicides—such as the vaginal contraceptive film or the vaginal inserts—come in packages small enough to carry easily in a purse or pocket for those times when you unexpectedly need pregnancy or disease protection and your partner does not use a condom.

IN A NUTSHELL

SPERMICIDES

Spermicides kill sperm and are good methods of birth control. The woman puts a spermicide in her vagina just before having sex. If used alone, spermicides are fairly effective in preventing pregnancy. A male condom and a spermicide together offer excellent protection against pregnancy and STDs, including AIDS. Spermicide gels also are added to a diaphragm or cervical cap to make them more effective.

Spermicides can be bought in drugstores without a prescription. They are available in several forms: foams, gels or jellies, suppositories (tablets), or dissolving film.

Spermicides can prevent gonorrhea and chlamydia, but it is not clear how much they protect against STDs that are caused by viruses, including AIDS.

Spermicides also can provide fairly good protection against pregnancy if you forget your birth control pills for several days in a row or do not refill the prescription in time. A condom plus spermicide is even better. An application of spermicide is a good addition to birth control methods like the cervical cap or condom. It is also a necessary part of using a diaphragm.

At any time, if your method develops a problem, like a condom tearing or your cervical cap being dislodged, an immediate application of spermicide may prevent conception. If such an accident should happen, in addition to adding spermicide, it is important to call your family planning practitioner about emergency medical contraception (see Chapter 16). Obviously, keeping a spermicide on hand is a good practice.

EFFECTIVENESS

For typical users, spermicides in any form, when used alone, have a first-year failure rate in protecting against pregnancy that ranges from 6 to 21 percent. Typical users are couples who do not use the spermicide every time they have sex or do not always use it correctly. Couples who use a spermicide every single time they have sex, and use it according to its directions, have the lowest failure rates. The rates are similar to those for condoms, diaphragms, and cervical caps.

SPERMICIDES AVAILABLE (1996)

Jellies and Gels
- Conceptrol Gel Disposables (pre-filled applicators)
- Koromex Jelly
- Koromex Crystal Clear Gel*
- Gynol II Original Formula* (no applicator included)
- Gynol II Extra Strength

Foams
- Koromex Foam
- Delfen Contraceptive Foam

Vaginal Suppositories
- Koromex Vaginal Inserts**
- Conceptrol Inserts**
- Semicid**
- Encare**

Contraceptive Film
- Vaginal Contraceptive Film (VCF)**

Bioadhesive Gel
- Advantage 24 (pre-filled applicators)

*To be used only with a diaphragm or condom; not to be used alone.
**Requires 10 to 15 minutes to melt before effective.

Highly important to the success of this method is placing the spermicide right at the cervix, which can be felt as a bump at the end of your vagina. Furthermore, some products require at least a 15-minute wait so they can melt and spread around before you have sex. However, spermicides are not all similar in how they should be used. For the greatest effectiveness, it is necessary to read the directions that come with each product.

Most spermicide failures are experienced by young women who are in their very fertile, peak reproductive years and by women who have intercourse frequently. The fewest failures occur with women whose risk of pregnancy is reduced because they have intercourse less often or are over age 35 and are not so fertile. But at all ages, the conscientious use of a spermicide improves its effectiveness as a birth control method.

SPERMICIDES AND DISEASE

In vaginal sex, spermicide users are clearly protected against the chlamydia and gonorrhea bacteria, which usually enter the body via the cervix. There is some evidence that they may also receive protection against cervical cancer and hepatitis B. Nonoxynol-9 kills the AIDS and herpes viruses in test tubes, but how effective it is against these diseases in actual use has not been determined. How well each product covers and protects every part of the vagina also is not known, although spermicidal foam appears to provide the most thorough coverage.

Family planning professionals advise that a male condom plus an application of spermicide, or a female condom used alone, seem to be the best protection against disease. Next in order of effectiveness are a condom used alone, a diaphragm or cervical cap used with spermicide, and a spermicide product used alone.

HEALTH EFFECTS

Spermicidal products cause very few side effects while providing good protection against pregnancy and a number of sexually transmitted diseases.

Beneficial Effects

As we noted above, spermicides are an effective destroyer of the viruses and bacteria that cause certain common STDs. Thus, they also seem to reduce the danger of acquiring pelvic inflammatory disease.

Irritations, Allergic Reactions, and Vaginitis

The most common health problem associated with spermicides is irritation involving the penis or the vagina. The symptoms generally

WHO SHOULD NOT DEPEND ON A SPERMICIDE?

Spermicides should not be used as the sole method of birth control by a woman who absolutely does not want to become pregnant. If you must avoid pregnancy for medical or other reasons, discuss with your family planning practitioner which contraceptive method or combination of methods could provide better protection.

are feelings of itching and burning. Sometimes these side effects disappear after a short period of use. If not, try another brand or type of spermicide, because the reaction may be to the amount of nonoxynol-9 or the perfume in the one you are using. To rule out either of these as a cause, try a product that is unscented or contains less nonoxynol-9.

When used very frequently—several times a day for many days—spermicides can irritate and crack the lining of the vagina, making it susceptible to disease organisms.

Nonoxynol-9 also can encourage the presence of candida albicans, the organism that causes yeast infections, because it kills bacteria that usually keep candidiasis under control in the vagina. If you have frequent yeast infections while using a contraceptive method that requires a spermicide, you may need to switch to one that does not involve its use. This is something to discuss with your health care provider.

A thorough review of all available data has led medical experts to conclude that the use of spermicides does not affect any pregnancy that may follow. Early reports of an association between the use of spermicides and spontaneous abortions or children born with birth defects did not hold up in recent studies.

SPERMICIDES AND HOW TO USE THEM

As we noted earlier, you can obtain a spermicide in a number of forms: aerosol foams, gels or jellies, vaginal inserts, and small squares of film that dissolve. Although all are easy to use, some are easier than others to carry with you in a pocket or purse.

Jellies, Gels, and Foams

Spermicides are available in a variety of foams, gels, and jellies. Starter packages of most brands contain the spermicide plus reusable applicators; refill packages and Ortho's Gynol II do not include applicators, which are necessary for using these spermicides. Products like Conceptrol Gel Disposables and Advantage 24 offer individual applicators prefilled with spermicide for one-time use.

Some products are made to be used primarily with the additional protection of a diaphragm or cervical cap. Others are formulated to be used alone, and an applicator of these generally will contain more nonoxynol-9 than an applicator of a product designed to accompany a diaphragm or condom. Read the label carefully to be sure you are getting the degree of protection you want.

Normal body temperature melts most spermicides, allowing them to spread around the vagina and over the opening of the cervix. Melting takes place within minutes, so these spermicides are effective almost immediately after application. For full protection, you must apply the spermicide high in the vagina, close to the cervix.

Most spermicides are effective for only 1 hour, so they should be applied not long before you have sex. If an hour passes before you have intercourse, add more spermicide. If you are going to have sex again and more than an hour has passed since you inserted spermicide, use another application.

The amount of active ingredient differs from product to product. It is important to use the applicator that comes with a particular spermicide, because the applicator is sized to provide the correct dose for its product only. To insert the applicator easily, choose a position that is comfortable for you. You can stand with a foot on a chair or bathtub, squat on your heels, or insert it while you are lying down.

Do not throw out the applicator when you have finished with that container of spermicide. Save it to use with refills. You will get more spermicide for your money if you buy refill containers that are sold without applicators.

After sex, do not douche or wash out the spermicide for at least 6 hours. A tampon or minipad used after lovemaking will protect you against any leakage.

For gels and jellies in tubes, remove the screw-on top of the tube and put on the applicator in its place. Squeeze the tube to fill the applicator until the plunger is pushed out completely. Unscrew the applicator, gently insert it deep into the vagina, and push in the plunger as far as it will go. Remove the applicator from the vagina by its barrel, not by the plunger. Pulling on the plunger may cause it to suction out some spermicide.

Contraceptive foams are available in pressurized aerosol cans and are used with applicators. Before using, it is important to shake the can thoroughly to mix the spermicide into the foam—the spermicide tends to settle in the bottom of the can. The foam should have the consistency of shaving cream—the more bubbles it has, the better it will spread around your vagina.

To fill the plunger-type plastic applicator, place it on the can of foam and either push or tilt it so foam flows into it. As the applicator fills, the foam pushes up the plunger. (The filling technique varies from brand to brand, and each package has directions explaining how to use it.) When full, insert the applicator deep into the vagina and push in the plunger until it stops. Remove the applicator with the plunger still pushed in to avoid withdrawing any foam. You can insert foam up to 30 minutes before you have sex. If you do not have sex within that time, add another applicator of foam just before you do have intercourse.

Care and Storage. Wash the applicator thoroughly inside and out with hot water and detergent or soap. Do not boil it, because the plastic is likely to melt. To keep it clean, store the applicator in the original box or in a closed plastic bag. Store all spermicides at room temperature, away from extreme heat or cold. They should not be used more than 2 years after purchase or beyond the expiration date marked on the package.

With foam, it is impossible to know how much remains in the

can after you have been using it a while. To make sure you do not run out, buy two containers at first and, from then on, buy another every time one becomes empty. That way you will always have a supply of foam on hand whenever you need it.

Cost. Gels and jellies cost about $10, depending on size and whether the package includes an applicator. Foams cost about $16 or more per can. After you have an applicator, it is more economical to buy the refill containers that are sold without applicators, because they offer more spermicide for the money.

Bioadhesive Gel

Newly available is a spermicide gel that combines nonoxynol-9 with a patented "bioadhesive" that clings to the cervix and the walls of the vagina for 24 hours. This product, Advantage 24, contains less nonoxynol-9 than many others—enough to protect against pregnancy but usually not enough to irritate the vagina or penis. It is not washed away by the man's ejaculate, the woman's menstruation, or any secretions. Advantage 24 is not perfumed or flavored and does not leak from the vagina. After it is applied, sex can take place anytime in the next 24 hours. One application, however, cannot be used for multiple acts of intercourse—additional applications are needed.

Advantage 24 is sold in prefilled applicators for one-time use. Before inserting it, you hold the thick end of the applicator and shake it vigorously—like a thermometer—to force the gel to the thin end. You then twist off the tab at the thin end, insert that end into your vagina as far as possible, and squeeze the thick end of the applicator to deposit the gel close to your cervix.

You can use Advantage 24 alone or with a condom. As with other spermicides, douching is not recommended. If you feel douching is necessary, wait at least 6 hours after your last intercourse.

Care and Storage. Store at room temperature, away from extreme heat and cold. For example, do not leave the package in a coat pocket or in a purse on a radiator.

Cost. Advantage 24 is sold in packages of three for $7.99 or six for $11.99.

Vaginal Suppositories (Inserts)

Vaginal suppositories (often called inserts) are pushed with a finger well up into the vagina, where they melt or foam, allowing the nonoxynol-9 to spread around the upper vagina and over the opening of the cervix. Depending on the brand, they must be inserted 10 or 15 minutes before sex and are effective for 1 hour. A new tablet is needed for every additional intercourse or if sex is delayed beyond the 1-hour time limit. As usual, it is best not to douche, but if you feel you must, do not douche until 6 hours have passed since your partner's last ejaculation.

The Encare suppository does not melt but instead foams as it dissolves. You may find that this foaming action creates a warm feeling in the vagina that feels strange at first.

Care and Storage. Keep suppositories away from extreme cold or heat and store at room temperature. If a tablet melts, leave it in its plastic casing in a cool place, such as the refrigerator, for about an hour, and it will regain its shape and firmness.

Cost. Suppositories range in price from about $8.99 for a dozen to $12 for 18. They are the least expensive of all spermicides, and the packages are small and easy to carry in a pocket or small purse.

Contraceptive Film

Vaginal contraceptive film (VCF) is a somewhat novel approach to using a spermicide. It can be used alone, but it is most effective when used with a condom or to back up a diaphragm or cervical cap, particularly during a woman's most fertile days. Each piece of film is 2 inches square, very thin and flexible. Like a vaginal suppository, it is pushed up as close to the cervix as possible. Body warmth melts the film, transforming it into a sperm-killing gel within 15 minutes. After it has melted, it is effective for 2 hours. If you want to have sex after that time, add a second piece of film. The gel washes away naturally after a few more hours have passed and leakage seldom is a problem.

To use vaginal contraceptive film, wash your hands and dry them well before you remove the film from its package. If your hands are damp, the film will stick to your fingers. Fold the square of VCF in half and then in half again. Find a comfortable position and use your longest finger to locate your cervix at the end of your vagina. Bend the folded VCF over your longest (middle) finger and hold it there with your thumb and forefinger as you push it into your vagina. Push the VCF up your vagina with your middle finger until the film reaches your cervix. You will know that it is in the right place when you can feel the bump of your cervix through the film. Insert the VCF quickly so it does not start to melt and stick to your finger. Practice a few times without having sex so you are able to put the film in quickly and correctly—all the way up to your cervix.

You can place VCF into your vagina up to 1 hour before you have sex. If you do not have intercourse within that time, however, you must use another VCF. Just remember to wait 15 minutes each time for it to melt and coat your cervix. Use a VCF for each intercourse. Afterwards, do not douche or wash out the VCF jelly for at least 6 hours. Because it dissolves so thoroughly, you probably will not feel the need to douche.

Care and Storage. VCF should be stored at room temperature. If kept in its sealed packet, VCF can be usable up to 4 years.

Cost. Vaginal contraceptive film is sold at prices that start at six for $7 or a dozen for $9.50.

PART TWO

Hormonal Methods

7

The Pill: Combined Oral Contraceptives

Birth control pills, also called oral contraceptives or OCs, offer almost complete protection against pregnancy when taken exactly as prescribed. They are available in several types and more than 20 different formulations. Most common are the "combination" pills, which contain synthetic versions of the two major female hormones: estrogen and progesterone. When combination pills originally became available, the dose of hormones was quite high; today much smaller amounts of hormones are used. In addition to the combination pill, there are progestin-only pills or "POPs," which are discussed in Chapter 8.

Combination pills come in three models: single phase, biphasic, and triphasic. All contain an estrogen and progestin (a synthetic form of progesterone), but the biphasic and triphasic pills provide these hormones in amounts that vary from one phase of the monthly cycle to another, in an effort to mimic a woman's natural hormonal cycle.

Birth control pills can be prescribed by physicians, nurse-midwives, nurse practitioners, and physician's assistants working in public and private clinics, HMOs, and other health care offices. "The

Pill" today is the most popular form of reversible contraception in the United States.

If you are under age 18 and wonder if the clinic or physician will tell your parents about your visit, you may find it helpful to ask some of the privacy questions listed on page 234 in Chapter 18.

NOTE: Contraceptive pills offer no protection against the AIDS virus and other sexually transmitted diseases.

During sex, a male condom used with a spermicide is the best protection against bacteria and viruses. A number of the women who use the Pill today also use condoms. A long-term, mutually faithful relationship or abstinence also makes it possible to avoid these diseases.

COMBINATION PILLS

As we explain in Chapter 1, the process of ovulation is directed by several hormones. These hormones act in a highly synchronized sequence every month, and the changes in their production by the body cause an egg to mature in one of the ovaries and then be released (ovulated). These changes in hormone production also cause the lining of the uterus to thicken with blood-rich tissue every month, in preparation for nurturing a fertilized egg.

All combination pills contain a synthetic estrogen and a synthetic progestin. They are taken for 3 consecutive weeks; during the fourth week either no pills or blank pills are taken, which causes a period of bleeding like a light menstruation. The Pill prevents pregnancy by means of several different mechanisms. The estrogen in the Pill suppresses certain other hormones that are necessary for ovulation. Without an egg, there can be no pregnancy. The progestin in the Pill causes the cervical mucus to remain thick and sticky, making it very difficult for sperm to get through the cervix to the uterus. It also helps suppress the hormones that govern ovulation.

IN A NUTSHELL

THE PILL

Combined birth control pills are taken by women. Each pill contains hormones, an estrogen and a progestin. These hormones cause changes in your body that prevent you from getting pregnant. The Pill is very effective in preventing pregnancy if it is taken every day about the same time.

The Pill does not protect you against STDs, including AIDS. For protection against disease, you or your partner need to use a condom as well.

You need a prescription from your doctor or a clinic such as Planned Parenthood to buy birth control pills. You can buy them from a drugstore or from the clinic. One pack of pills will last for 1 month. Your doctor or nurse will tell you when to take the first one. The last seven pills are a different color and you will get your period for a few days while taking them. You start the next pack of pills as soon as the first pack is finished.

If you take the Pill you should not smoke, because you increase your risk of a heart attack, stroke, or clots in your blood vessels, even if you are a young woman.

When some women use the Pill, they have mild side effects such as gaining a few pounds, nausea, headaches, bleeding a little between periods, breast tenderness, and acne. If these bother you, tell the nurse or doctor who prescribed the Pill.

It is unusual to have serious side effects, but if you do, call your nurse or doctor right away. These serious effects may be signalled by abdominal pain, very bad headaches, unusual pain in your legs, chest pain, eye problems like blurred vision, or difficulty breathing.

The combination pill is one of the most effective of the reversible methods of birth control available today. There are definite advantages to pills that contain both hormones. The estrogen helps to stabilize the lining of the uterus—the endometrium—so it is less likely to shed between menstrual cycles and cause breakthrough bleeding or spotting. The progestin produces thick cervical mucus that prevents sperm from penetrating, may inhibit ovulation, and alters the lining of the uterus so that it prevents the implantation of a fertilized egg. Both hormones provide some important health benefits, described later in this chapter.

Over the years, changes have been made in the amounts of estrogen and progestin in the Pill. Almost all oral contraceptives now contain greatly reduced levels of both hormones, making them even safer to use.

The Biphasic Pill

The first phased oral contraceptive, Ortho-Novum 10/11, was two-phased (biphasic). With biphasic contraceptives, the pills taken for the first 10 days of the month each contain 0.5 milligram of progestin, and the last 11 pills in the cycle contain 1.0 milligram. The estrogen dose remains steady throughout the cycle at 35 micrograms.

The Triphasic Pill

The successful introduction of the biphasic pill some years ago led to the development of the triphasic formula. In the triphasic pill, the amounts of both the synthetic estrogen and progestin change during the month. Although phasic pills are promoted as mimicking a woman's natural hormone cycle, not even the manufacturers are sure this makes any difference. The various brands take different approaches to doing this. One product, Ortho-Novum 7/7/7, for instance, uses the same amount of estrogen throughout the month but the amount of progestin changes every 7 days. Two other brands, Triphasil and Tri-Levlen, use a somewhat more potent form of synthetic progestin, and the dose levels change with each phase. The level of estrogen in these two brands also changes from phase to phase. Phases are indicated by different pill colors.

Because each brand of triphasic pills takes a different approach to imitating natural hormone cycles, some experts wonder about the validity of such efforts. If the manufacturers of oral contraceptives were truly trying to copy a woman's natural cycle, these critics point out, all brands of triphasics would follow a single pattern.

Regardless of their individual approaches, the total amounts of estrogen and progestin that phasic pills provide over the course of a month is only a little less than the amount in a month's supply of any low-dose, single-phase, combination pill. All combination pills prevent ovulation and alter the cervical mucus and endometrium, and there is little difference in their effectiveness.

Triphasic pills do have one small drawback. The three phases of different-colored pills sometimes can be difficult to figure out or remember, especially if you are new to oral contraceptives.

HOW EFFECTIVE IS THE PILL?

When taken every day, an oral contraceptive that combines an estrogen and a progestin is extremely effective. In perfect use, a pill that contains at least 30 micrograms of estrogen has about a 1 to 2 percent failure rate. Pills containing 20 micrograms of estrogen have a failure rate of 2 percent.

Among typical users, who may forget a pill occasionally, oral contraception is slightly less effective. Studies of typical users of combination pills reveal a failure rate of up to 3 percent during the first year of use. The effectiveness of an oral contraceptive depends almost entirely on how consistently the pills are taken.

IS THE PILL FOR YOU?

If you have difficulty following instructions or keeping to a schedule, the Pill may be a bad choice for you. If you are coping with a severe depression or a major psychiatric illness, a drug or alcohol dependency, or if you have a history of taking medications incorrectly, other methods may be a better match. Talk to a health care provider—most of them are trained to find the best method for the user.

HOW REVERSIBLE IS THE PILL?

Generally speaking, if you are fertile before you begin using the Pill, your basic ability to conceive will not be affected by this method. Many women become pregnant within a few months after they stopped taking the Pill; for a substantial percentage of women, conception may take 6 months to a year and sometimes longer. This is

AVAILABLE ORAL CONTRACEPTIVES (1996)

Product	Manufacturer
CONSTANT-DOSE ORAL CONTRACEPTIVES	
Alesse	Wyeth-Ayerst
Brevicon	Roche
Demulen 1/35	Searle
Desogen	Organon
Levlen	Berlex
Lo-Ovral	Wyeth-Ayerst
Modicon	Ortho
Nordette	Wyeth-Ayerst
Norinyl 1+35	Roche
Ortho-Cept	Ortho
Ortho-Cyclen	Ortho
Ortho-Novum 1/35	Ortho
Ovcon 35	Bristol-Myers Squibb
PHASIC ORAL CONTRACEPTIVES (Except for Desogen, all these products come in 21-day and 28-day packs. A 28-day pack has seven blank pills.)	
Ortho-Novum 7/7/7	Ortho
Ortho-Novum 10/11	Ortho
Ortho Tri-Cyclen	Ortho
Tri-Levlen	Berlex
Tri-Norinyl	Roche
Triphasil	Wyeth-Ayerst
ORAL CONTRACEPTIVES WITH 50 μg OF ESTROGEN (not usually recommended)	
Demulen 1/50	Searle
Norinyl 1+50	Roche
Ortho-Novum 1/50	Ortho
Ovcon 50	Bristol-Myers Squibb
Ovral	Wyeth-Ayerst

(Source: Physicians' Desk Reference, 1996, p. 210)

not very different from the length of time it can take for some women who have not used birth control pills. How long a woman was on the Pill does not appear to affect her return to fertility.

In fact, an inability to conceive does not appear to be related to the Pill itself. Instead, any infertility after pill use is usually due to the woman's age, a physical condition that might have been in existence before she started this method, or problems that may have developed independent of the Pill during its use.

HEALTH EFFECTS

Oral contraceptives have benefits in addition to providing excellent birth control. They protect you against cancer of the ovaries and the endometrium, ovarian cysts, and benign breast lumps. They regularize menstrual cycles and relieve many problems associated with menstruation, such as severe cramps and heavy bleeding.

On the other hand, the Pill may cause some side effects. If you have heart or blood vessel problems, a combined oral contraceptive may not be the best hormonal method for you; instead you may be able to safely use a progestin-only method. Virtually all the research on long-term complications of oral contraceptives was based on the earlier Pills that contained high doses of estrogen and progestin. The few short-term studies of the newer Pills suggest that cardiovascular side effects have declined now that hormone doses are lower.

What has not changed, however, is the dangerous interaction between a combined oral contraceptive and smoking, especially if you are over age 35. If you use the Pill, you should try not to smoke.

The Pill's Benefits

The Pill has protective effects against some common disorders:

- benign breast disease (fibrocystic disease)
- cancer of the ovaries
- cancer of the endometrium
- functional cysts on the ovaries
- iron deficiency anemia caused by heavy menstruation

- pelvic inflammatory disease
- pregnancy in the fallopian tubes (ectopic pregnancy)
- irregular menstrual cycles

Almost all the studies demonstrating these protective effects were conducted with women who had used high-dose oral contraceptives for many years. Although long-term studies of lower-dose pills are not yet available, it seems likely that similar benefits—and fewer side effects—are associated with low-dose pills.

Benign breast disease is less likely. Also known as fibrocystic disease, this is the most common cause of a noncancerous breast lump. The breast feels lumpy and may be tender in the days just before a menstrual period. Women who take birth control pills are less likely to have fibrocystic disease. It is found least often in women who take pills with larger amounts of progestin. This protection increases with every year that the Pill is used and persists for at least a year after it is discontinued.

Protection against ovarian and endometrial cancers. The Pill reduces a woman's risk of cancer of the ovaries or cancer of the endometrium (the lining of the uterus).

Ovarian cancer is the fourth leading cause of cancer deaths in women. It is particularly worrisome because it usually produces no symptoms until it is far advanced. It is fatal for almost 80 percent of the women who develop it. Ovarian cancer is thought to be associated with long stretches of ovulation that are not interrupted by pregnancy and breastfeeding. This cancer is more common today than when women were pregnant frequently and routinely breastfed their children, which meant they did not ovulate for long periods. The Pill may protect against cancer of the ovaries because it stops ovulation. The risk of ovarian cancer in women who ever used the Pill (most of which were higher dose pills) was found to be reduced by 30 to 70 percent. The longer the use, the greater the protection.

Cancer of the endometrium is also a common disease. The risk of endometrial cancer in women who have used the Pill for at least 2 years is about 40 percent less than among women who have never

THE PILL AND SICKLE CELL DISEASE

One of the widely held misconceptions about oral contraceptives is that they cannot be used by a woman who has sickle cell disease, an inherited, chronic, severe anemia. Research has demonstrated that women with sickle cell anemia who take the Pill are not more vulnerable to the sickle crises that occur when the sickle-shaped blood cells block small blood vessels. In fact, the Pill is an excellent contraceptive for these women, for whom pregnancy is dangerous. And even better than the combination pill is the progestin-only pill.

used combined oral contraceptives. The longer a woman uses the Pill, the greater her protection against this cancer.

Fewer functional ovarian cysts. During the menstrual cycle, some ovarian follicles respond to hormone stimulation by continuing to grow instead of bursting open and releasing an egg or simply disappearing at the end of the cycle. These become functional cysts. "Functional" means the cyst is not due to disease but results from the function of the normal cycle. Many times there are no symptoms, but some cysts cause a variety of problems, including abdominal pain, pain during sex, and menstrual difficulties, including delayed menstruation. In three epidemiological studies, the risk of functional ovarian cysts was reduced by the use of birth control pills, probably because the Pill suppresses the normal hormone cycle that stimulates ovulation. In a British study, use of the Pill led to a 64 percent drop in the incidence of these cysts.

Fewer cases of iron deficiency anemia. Iron is essential to the production of hemoglobin, that part of the red blood cell that transports oxygen from the lungs to the rest of the body, where oxygen fuels vital chemical reactions. If a women does not get enough iron in her diet or loses it because of heavy menstruation, she may develop iron deficiency anemia. If this becomes substantial, it can cause a feeling of being tired all the time. Severe forms lead to dizziness, breathing difficulties during physical effort, and angina.

Combined oral contraceptives inhibit the normal development cycle of the lining of the uterus, during which the uterine lining grows rich with extra blood in preparation for the implanting of a fertilized egg. When this does not occur, the amount of monthly bleeding is considerably diminished. Pill users seldom have the heavy periods that are a common cause of iron deficiency anemia in women.

Less chance of pelvic inflammatory disease. About one million women in the United States experience episodes of pelvic inflammatory disease (PID) every year. PID refers to infection in the upper part of the reproductive tract and often follows a sexually transmitted disease. Certain common STDs, such as chlamydia and gonorrhea (the most frequent causes of PID), produce few or no symptoms in the lower genital tract. If not treated, however, they can spread upward through the rest of the reproductive system, causing PID, damaging the fallopian tubes, and leaving scar tissue behind. Every bout of PID does additional damage, greatly increasing a woman's chance of being infertile or having an ectopic pregnancy, a pregnancy that grows in her tubes instead of her uterus.

A major U.S. study of PID in users of oral contraceptives indicated that women who had ever used the Pill had one-half the risk of PID, compared to women their age who did not use oral contraceptives. If a woman were on the Pill for at least 1 year, her risk was reduced by 70 percent. Although the actual mechanism for this protection is not known, researchers believe the thickening of the cervical mucus that occurs during Pill use probably prevents infectious organisms from entering the upper reproductive system. Because the Pill can also shorten menstrual periods and reduce blood flow, the disease organisms that find it easier to enter the sytem during bleeding have less opportunity to do so.

NOTE: Although the Pill appears to protect the upper reproductive system, it offers the lower part of the system—the vagina and cervix—no protection from the microbes that cause herpes, gonorrhea, genital warts, chlamydia, or syphilis. Nor does it protect against hepatitis B or AIDS.

Reduced risk of an ectopic pregnancy. When a pregnancy develops outside the uterus, usually in a fallopian tube, it is called an *ectopic*, or out-of-place, pregnancy. Currently, about 1 in every 100 pregnancies in the United States is ectopic. These pregnancies are more common in women whose tubes are abnormal or blocked by scar tissue. Sperm may get past the blockage and fertilize an egg, but the egg may implant in the fallopian tube if it is hindered from moving normally toward the uterus. Because the Pill stops ovulation, the chance of an ectopic pregnancy is greatly reduced.

Menstrual cycle benefits. The Pill provides a number of menstrual cycle improvements. It lessens cramps, can shorten the number of days of bleeding, and reduces the amount of blood lost. It improves cycle regularity and decreases the pain some women feel at ovulation. Some women's premenstrual symptoms, including depression and tension, are diminished as well. These effects are especially helpful for women who suffer from premenstrual syndrome and for teenagers who experience difficult and painful periods that interfere with school and other activities.

Other benefits. In addition to the health benefits that the Pill may provide in its role as a contraceptive, it can also be used solely as therapy for several disorders, including dysfunctional uterine bleeding (bleeding that is not normal or cyclical), painful periods, acne, excessive body hair, and endometriosis.

In endometriosis, fragments of the tissue that normally lines the uterus migrate and grow in other places. The fallopian tubes, ovaries, intestines, surface of the bladder, and pelvic wall may be affected. The tissue continues to respond to the menstrual cycle and bleeds each month. Not surprisingly, endometriosis causes considerable pain, especially during menstruation, and can interfere with the normal functioning of the ovaries and fallopian tubes. By reducing the monthly thickening and shedding of the endometrium, oral contraceptives can be an effective treatment for this condition.

FOR THE WOMAN OVER AGE 35

Most experts in family planning feel that healthy, nonsmoking women can use low-dose oral contraceptives until menopause. "Healthy" generally means a woman with no high blood pressure, cardiovascular disease, high blood cholesterol, diabetes, or obesity. Many physicians argue that not only are birth control pills safe for women over age 35, but certain of the Pill's health benefits may have more value as a woman gets older.

A number of obstetricians and gynecologists now believe women should stay on the Pill well into their forties, because the Pill's estrogen will make up for the drop in natural estrogen production that takes place at this time. Maintaining good estrogen levels protects a mature woman against bone thinning and heart disease.

The Pill's Possible Risks

Estrogens and progestins affect many systems in the body, not just the reproductive tract. Anyone taking an oral contraceptive should be aware of possible complications and the symptoms of those complications. When taking the Pill, you should discuss with your health care provider any physical or emotional changes you notice that may be the result of Pill use.

Slightly greater risk of cardiovascular diseases, including thrombophlebitis and blood clots. The most serious complications linked to the Pill since the earliest studies are those of the heart and blood vessels. The risk is increased if you smoke. Severe heart and blood vessel problems, however, are rare in women who take the new low-dose pills and do not smoke.

The formation of blood clots in the veins, particularly in the legs, is perhaps the most common cardiovascular effect, although it does not occur very often. The danger of such clots is that they can break off, get stuck somewhere in the blood system, and block the blood supply to an important organ like the heart, brain, lungs, or eyes. A blood clot usually has no symptoms until it hinders blood flow at some point in the body. It then will affect the function of that organ or tissue and also cause severe pain.

Thrombophlebitis is the inflammation of part of a vein. Its symptoms are swelling, redness, and sensitivity to touch along the course of the involved vein. It also occurs only rarely.

There has been a marked, overall decline in the percentage of women having heart attacks or blood clots associated with taking the Pill. And women who are taking the current low-dose pills are at no greater risk of stroke than women who do not use the Pill, according to a study published in 1996.

NOTE: A woman who wants to use even the low-dose pills should stop smoking, regardless of her age. The risk of heart attack is increased nearly twelvefold in women who smoke. When women smoke and take the Pill, the risk of heart attack increases fiftyfold.

In late 1995, a European study suggested that women who used a combination pill that contained the very new progestins, desogestrel and gestodene, had a greater risk of blood clots than did the users of pills containing older progestins. The reported risk was 30 instances of blood clots in 100,000 women who used these pills. (Just by being pregnant, women have a blood clot risk of 60 per 100,000.) More recent studies have disputed this report.

A WORD OF CAUTION

When a report appears in the media about a newly discovered danger associated with the Pill—or any other method—it is often exaggerated. It is important not to panic but to continue using your contraceptive until you and your doctor have had a chance to learn more about the particular study and whether it applies to you. Unless you want to get pregnant, it is important not to stop using a contraceptive even for a short time. Keeping another birth control method on hand as a backup, and learning to use it, is wise.

Two U.S. brands contain desogestrel: Desogen, made by Organon, and Ortho-Cept, made by Ortho. Pills with gestodene are not sold in the United States. If you are using Desogen or Ortho-Cept, you may want to discuss this study with your health care provider.

Diabetes. If you have diabetes but you are healthy otherwise, you may be able to use the Pill, although some experimentation may be necessary to find a Pill formula that does not aggravate the diabetes.

Blood pressure may rise in some women. Both estrogens and progestins may affect blood pressure, and hypertension was associated with earlier Pills. Today, however, it is uncommon in women who take low-dose oral contraceptives. Blood pressure levels may rise slightly in some women but, when the pills are stopped, will drop to former levels in a few weeks. It is wise to have your blood pressure checked periodically after you start any type of drug. If you have a strong family history of early hypertension or have experienced a rise in blood pressure during pregnancy, you should inform your health care provider. In this circumstance, you should be diligent in having your blood pressure checked regularly. If it rises, your provider may suggest a pill with a different formula, or a "minipill" that contains only progestin, or another birth control method entirely.

Possible slight increase in breast cancer risk. A recent, worldwide study of 53,297 women with breast cancer and 100,239 women without this disease concluded that there is a small increase in the risk of breast cancer while women are taking the combined pill or if they have used this method in the past 10 years. There is no evidence of an increase in the risk of having breast cancer diagnosed 10 or more years after stopping the Pill. Women who take a combined oral contraceptive and also have a strong family history of breast cancer, small breast lumps, or abnormal mammograms should always be followed carefully by their physicians.

Possible slight increase in risk of cervical dysplasia. Studies show that women who use oral contraceptives may be at a slightly increased risk of developing cervical dysplasia (abnormal cell changes in the cervix) and cervical cancer. The Pill does not worsen existing dysplasia, however. Even without taking the Pill, any woman who has multiple sexual partners is at increased risk for cervical cancer. The disease is more likely to develop in women who smoke.

It should be noted that mild dysplasia may clear up on its own; more severe dysplasia, which often precedes cervical cancer, can be treated and cured if detected early and treated promptly. An annual Pap test finds almost all cases of dysplasia, usually long before the cell changes develop into cancer. It is important for women who take the Pill, who have many sex partners, and who smoke to have regular Pap tests.

Slight increase in chlamydial cervicitis. Birth control pills can cause a condition in which the cells that usually line the inside of the cervical canal migrate out and around the mouth of the cervix. These migrating cells are more vulnerable to chlamydial infections. The increase in infections, however, is not accompanied by an increase in pelvic inflammatory disease (PID), which often is associated with chlamydia. It is possible that the progestin in the Pill thickens the cervical mucus so the chlamydial organisms are less able to get up into the reproductive tract and damage the fallopian tubes.

Gallbladder disease may develop in certain women. The Pill may accelerate the development of gallbladder disease in women who are already susceptible. Symptoms of gallbladder problems, including gallstones, range from fever and abdominal tenderness to severe pain. Indigestion that is made worse by eating fatty foods also is linked to gallstones.

Common Complaints or Side Effects

The advent of oral contraceptives with a lower dose of hormones has reduced the number of side effects. In general, minor side effects subside after a few months. If you think you are experiencing a side effect and it persists longer than three months, talk to your practitioner about switching to a different pill. *Continue taking the pills you have, however, until the prescription is changed or you start another contraceptive method.*

Nausea. Although nausea is not a common problem with low-dose pills, it does still occur, usually during the first month or the first few days of each new pack of pills. It seldom causes vomiting. Many women find they can reduce nausea by taking the Pill at bedtime, with a meal, or with an evening snack. If nausea occurs for the first time after months or years of being on the Pill, and cannot be attributed to flu or some other infection, it may be a sign of pregnancy.

Headaches. While taking the Pill, some women develop severe, long-lasting, or recurrent headaches. Women who are prone to migraines may notice an increase in their severity. There is no solid evidence, however, that the Pill increases the frequency of migraines. If your headaches are severe, persistent, and accompanied by vision disturbances, discuss them with your health care provider. You may want to use another form of contraception. If you have occasional migraines that are not too severe, a Pill with less estrogen is less likely to intensify them.

Breast Swelling. Breast swelling is an effect of estrogen that women often experience naturally during their monthly cycle. Low-dose pills seldom cause such swelling so, if it does occur, it is more likely to be a sign of pregnancy.

Fluid Retention. Oral contraceptives occasionally may cause you to retain fluid, resulting in swollen fingers and ankles. Bring this to the attention of your health care provider.

Weight Gain. The progestin in the Pill can cause an increase in appetite and consequent slight weight gain—but it is seldom more than 2 to 4 pounds.

Depression. A large-scale British study in 1985 reported no difference in the incidence of depression among women who were on the Pill and women who used other forms of birth control. Women with a history of depression or mental illness, however, are more likely to experience a worsening of their symptoms while on the Pill.

Interest in Sex. Conflicting reports exist about the effect of the birth control pill on sexual desire. Some Pill users say that their interest in sex diminishes and others find they enjoy sex more because they are no longer afraid of getting pregnant. A few have less vaginal lubrication when they are aroused, which can make sex uncomfortable unless it is remedied by adding a lubricant to the vagina.

Breastfeeding Problems. The combined Pill diminishes milk production and is not recommended when a woman is nursing. In addition, the hormones pass into the milk in small amounts. If you really want to use an oral contraceptive while breastfeeding, you should use a progestin-only pill instead, which will not reduce the supply of breast milk. (See Chapter 17 for more information on breastfeeding and contraceptive use.)

Vision Problems. Double vision, loss of vision, eye pain or swelling, or discomfort while wearing contact lenses are rare side effects of the Pill. If any of these symptoms occurs, you should stop taking the Pill, use another method, and talk with your physician.

Skin Changes. Sometimes a faint, brownish discoloration appears on the cheekbones, forehead, and upper lip when the Pill is being used, and this "mask" will be intensified by sunlight. Known as chloasma or melasma, this masklike effect usually fades in a few months or so if the Pill is discontinued, although in some women it does become permanent.

Menstrual Disturbances

Scanty or Missed Periods. The monthly increase of blood and tissue in the lining of the uterus is almost always reduced when you take birth control pills. As a result, the amount of blood lost every month is less. It is rare, however, for no bleeding to occur during the days the Pill is not taken. If this happens, you should contact your health care provider—it may be a sign of pregnancy.

Breakthrough Bleeding or Spotting. When vaginal bleeding or staining occurs between periods, it is called breakthrough bleeding. This happens more often among women on very low dose pills, on progestin-only pills, or on other progestin-only methods. It is more an annoyance than a medical problem. Most breakthrough bleeding occurs during the first months on the Pill. Low estrogen causes the lining of the uterus (endometrium) to become so thin it breaks loose from the uterus at unexpected times. With low-dose pills or progestin-only methods, such bleeding can be caused by missing a single pill or by not taking a pill at the same time every day. If the bleeding occurs in more than one cycle and lasts for more than a few days, talk to your practitioner.

Breakthrough bleeding also can appear after you have been on the Pill for a long time. If it occurs early in your cycle, your practitioner may prescribe a small amount of extra estrogen to stop it. If it occurs later, a pill with a stronger form of progestin might be prescribed, to give extra support to the endometrium.

Before your practitioner decides what to do, you should have a physical examination to rule out other possible causes of abnormal bleeding, such as a benign growth or a cancer. If the exam, including a Pap test, reveals no other possible reason for the bleeding, you could switch to a higher dose pill or another method, or you may be able to ignore the bleeding, if it is light and minor.

Early Menstruation. Another form of breakthrough bleeding is menstruation that begins a day or two before you stop taking the monthly schedule of active pills. Continue to take your pills on schedule. If this happens often, check with your health care provider, who may suggest you take a brand with extra estrogen so the endometrium does not shed prematurely.

NOTE: Changing brands may eliminate or reduce annoying side effects. One advantage of using oral contraceptives is that there are many different formulations available. You can try pills with different amounts of estrogen or a different type of progestin to find one that suits you best.

Other Cautions

Because the Pill can be associated with an increased risk of blood clots, it is best to stop birth control pills for three or four weeks before surgery, although this risk has diminished with the low-dose pills.

Because you are more prone to develop blood clots right after childbirth, you shouldn't take the Pill until 14 days after delivery. Unless you are nursing, however, start birth control on or soon after that day—it is possible to ovulate very soon after giving birth. If you are breastfeeding, do not use the combined Pill. If you want an oral contraceptive, use a progestin-only pill. (Chapter 8 describes progestin-only pills; Chapter 17 discusses breastfeeding and contraception.)

If you take oral contraceptives after you unknowingly have become pregnant, the risk of your child having any abnormality will not increase above the usual 5 to 6 percent risk that exists for all pregnancies.

If you develop new physical changes such as breast swelling and nausea after using the Pill for some time, you should suspect pregnancy. Talk to your health care provider immediately.

GETTING AND USING THE COMBINATION PILL

A visit to a clinic or a doctor is necessary if you are interested in using the Pill, because oral contraceptives are only sold by prescription. To determine if you are a good candidate for this birth control method, the health care provider will take your personal and family medical history, perform a physical and a pelvic examination, and arrange for any needed lab tests. After the test results are in, if you are considered a good candidate for the Pill, you will be given a prescription for birth control pills. You can fill the prescription at your health center or at any drugstore. One pack of pills lasts 1 month. Many providers prescribe 6 to 12 month supplies of pills to women who have used pills before. (It is not necessary to buy more than one or two packs at a time.)

All but one brand of the Pill are available in either a 21-day or 28-day supply. If you choose the 21-day program, you will stop taking pills for 7 days and then start a new packet. If it is a 28-day pack, the last seven pills are "blanks"—they have no active ingredients. You begin the next pack after finishing the last one. For many women, taking a pill every day lessens the chance of forgetting to start again. If you think there is a chance you might forget to start up again after a week of not taking pills, use the 28-day program. With either pack of pills, you will begin menstruating in the days immediately following the last *active* pill.

Choose a backup method of birth control. Condoms, vaginal film, or a foam spermicide are reasonably effective, easy-to-use methods. Keep one of these backup methods handy in case you forget to take a pill, forget to buy more, or stop taking them for any reason. If you may need STD protection, condoms are a good choice.

Choose the best day of the month for starting your pills. To use a combined oral contraceptive successfully, it is vital that you take it every day around the same time, without fail, so you maintain an effective level of the hormones in your body. For this reason, you want to make your pill-taking as easy as possible to remember. You also will need to remember to buy the next pack before your supply runs out. Whichever day you choose for starting your pills from then on will be the day you begin every new pill packet. Health care providers and the manufacturers of oral contraceptives usually suggest starting your pill packet on a Sunday, or on the first day of your menstrual period. Read the package insert for instructions for your particular brand. If you begin your first pack of pills on a Sunday, you will start every subsequent packet on a Sunday.

Link your pill-taking to another daily activity. It will be easier to remember to take a birth control pill at the same time every day if you associate it with something you usually do without fail, such as brushing your teeth or preparing for bed. Pill packages are designed to indicate whether you have taken that day's pill.

To avoid the possibility of nausea, do not take the pill on an empty stomach. Take your pill after dinner or with a bedtime snack.

Begin the next packet of pills on time or you might ovulate—and you could become pregnant. If you are using 21-day packs and extend the pill-free interval beyond the seventh day, there is a chance you might ovulate during your next cycle. If you are using a 28-pill pack and do not start a new pack the day after you finish the old one, you also put yourself at risk of ovulating, because the last seven pills contain no active ingredients.

During the 7 hormone-free days, the other hormones in your body that stimulate ovulation gradually return to almost normal levels, enabling the ovary to function again. If you lengthen the hormone-free interval at all, by missing a pill at either end of the interval, the ovary may release a mature egg a few days after the interval. When on oral contraceptives, the highest fertility is after the hormone-free period, not at mid-month. Furthermore, the effect of the pill on the cervical mucus will be at its lowest, so adding to the hormone-free days can allow sperm to pass through the cervix.

NOTE: Missing a pill just before or just after the hormone-free interval is riskier than missing a pill in the middle of your cycle.

After the interval of no active pills or no pills at all (depending on whether you use a 28-day or 21-day pack), the first seven active pills restore the ovaries to a non-active state.

WHAT TO DO IF YOU FORGET TO TAKE A COMBINATION PILL

If you miss taking one pill, take the delayed pill at once—and continue to take the rest of the pills as usual.

If you miss two active tablets in Week One or Week Two, you should take two tablets the day you remember and two tablets the next day. Then take one tablet a day until you have finished the pack. If you have sex during the 7 days following the missing pills, use your backup method.

If you miss two active tablets in Week Three, or you miss three or more active tablets in a row, throw out the rest of the pack and start a new one the same day. Use a backup method if you have sex in the 7 days after you have missed the pills.

If you are using a 28-day pack and forget to take any nonactive pills (the last seven), throw away the missed pills and continue to finish the packet on schedule. Forgetting the non-active pills does not increase your risk of pregnancy. Be sure to start your next pack on time, however.

If you continue to forget to take your pills, this may not be the best method for you. Think hard about your temperament and lifestyle. Other contraceptive methods—like Norplant or Depo-Provera injections—may better match your particular needs.

Keep an extra package of pills on hand at all times. If you misplace your packet or forget to have your prescription refilled, you will not run the risk of missing a pill if you have a second pack. Furthermore, if you get the flu or some other illness that causes vomiting, you need to take extra pills to replace those that do not remain in your stomach.

When you start your pills dictates when you have your period. Your menstrual period will usually occur sometime during the last 7 days of a cycle—after you finish the *active* pills. You may bleed for only a couple of days or only have some spotting. The blood also may be brownish in color.

If you miss one menstrual period, but have taken your pills at the same time and every day, it does not mean you are pregnant. It is possible to miss a period now and then while on the Pill. If you are concerned, call your health care provider.

If you miss two menstrual periods in a row despite taking your birth control pills at the same time every day, you may be pregnant. Call your doctor or clinic for an early pregnancy test immediately.

If you do not menstruate and have forgotten to take one or more pills during that cycle, your chances of being pregnant are greater. Do not start a new pack of tablets. Instead, use another form of contraception and contact your clinic or doctor for an early pregnancy test. The early tests available today, which measure the pregnancy hormone, human chorionic gonadotropin, in the blood, can provide reliable results as early as one week after conception. The tests sold in drugstores are not sensitive enough to be positive this early.

HOW TO HANDLE SIDE EFFECTS

Vomiting or Diarrhea

Vomiting right after taking a pill prevents the hormones from being absorbed. If vomiting happens within two hours after you have swallowed a tablet, take another one as soon as you can. (If you use up all your active pills, take the pill for that day from your extra packet.) If you cannot keep a pill down for a second day, which may happen during a severe bout of flu, use your backup method until you have been back on the pills for 7 days or have had your next period. Then start a new package of pills on your usual day, even if you are bleeding. If you have severe diarrhea for more than one day, also use your backup method for the rest of the month and then begin another cycle of pills as usual.

Do not use the pill packet you have "borrowed" pills from because it will not have enough left. Save it—you may need to use it for extra pills sometime again. To avoid confusion, label it "Extra Pills."

Drug Interactions

The effectiveness of the Pill can be weakened by a number of prescription drugs. Drugs that may affect the performance of the Pill include some medications for treating tuberculosis, drugs for controlling seizures, and certain prescription drugs for headaches.

Certain classes of drugs stimulate the liver to greater activity, causing it to process other chemicals—like birth control pills—faster, diminishing their effect. Such liver-stimulating drugs include the antiseizure medicines used to treat epilepsy that contain phenylbutazone (Butazolidin), phenobarbital, phenytoin (Dilantin), primidone (Mysoline), and carbamazepine (Tegretol). If you must take any of these, it probably would be prudent to use a different type of birth control. The possibility of such an interaction is something to discuss with your physician and pharmacist. Newer anticonvulsants may not have this effect.

A type of barbiturate called butalbital, found in prescription headache tablets such as Fiorinal, Fioricet, Esgic, and others, also decreases the effectiveness of hormonal contraceptives. It might be wise to use backup protection if you need these painkillers for more than one day.

The tuberculosis antibiotic rifampin and oral antifungal medications containing griseofulvin (Fulvicin, Grifulvin V) could reduce the effectiveness of the Pill. Griseofulvin increases menstrual irregularities for women using oral contraceptives. You may want to use another birth control method while you are using these drugs.

Obviously, whenever a new medicine is prescribed for you, or a blood test is scheduled, you should remind your caregiver that you are taking birth control pills. It is also a good idea to remind your pharmacist. Because pharmacists are drug specialists, they may be more up-to-date on possible interactions between new drugs and the Pill.

COST

The cost of using oral contraceptives includes having a physical examination when the Pill is prescribed for the first time and at regular intervals thereafter while you continue to use this method. Physicals range from $60 to $175, plus charges for the necessary laboratory tests. The cost depends on whether you go to a government-funded clinic, a health maintenance organization (HMO), a private physician, a private health care facility, or a Planned Parenthood or other women's health center. Clinics supported by government agencies may charge a sliding fee, which usually means you pay according to your income. You can compare prices charged for the examination by telephoning health centers and doctors' offices.

The cost of filling a prescription for the Pill may range from $17 to $25 for a month's supply, depending on the type and brand of pill and the pharmacy filling the prescription. Since there are 13 menstrual cycles in each year, the expense of birth control pills for one year can range from $221 to $325. Packets of pills cost less if you buy them from large drugstore chains or from nonprofit or publicly funded clinics.

The majority of HMOs require only their usual co-payment charge ($5 to $20) for the necessary physical examination and for filling the prescription every month. In some states, birth control expenses are reimbursed in part by Medicaid. Some, but not many, conventional health insurance plans may cover the expense of oral contraceptives.

8

The Pill: Progestin-Only Pills (POPs)

Progestin-only pills (POPs) are variants of the more commonly used combined (estrogen and progestin) oral contraceptives. Because POPs have no estrogen and only very small amounts of progestin, they are sometimes called "minipills." Like Depo-Provera and Norplant, POPs do not contain the estrogen thought to lead to serious cardiovascular complications, such as blood clots and thrombophlebitis. They also are thought to be safer than the combined pill for women who smoke. A POP is taken every day of the month, even during menstrual periods. It can be started as early as a week after childbirth or immediately after a miscarriage or abortion.

This birth control pill protects against pregnancy four ways: (1) Its chief impact is the thickening of the cervical mucus, thus stopping sperm from entering the uterus. (2) It suppresses ovulation in about half the women who use it. (3) It slows the movement of an egg through the fallopian tubes. (4) It causes the lining of the uterus to become inhospitable to a fertilized egg. Making the cervical mucus difficult for sperm to penetrate is the minipill's most immediate and useful effect; the other actions chiefly enhance its effectiveness.

EFFECTIVENESS AND REVERSIBILITY

The progestin-only pill needs to be taken on a strict schedule. The possibility of getting pregnant returns faster with this pill than it does with the combination pill.

Failure Rate

The failure rate of the POP ranges from 0.5 percent for women who use it perfectly to 5 percent for women who sometimes take the pill late or forget it. Women who are less fertile because they are older or are breastfeeding have the least chance of pregnancy while using this pill.

With this pill, *any* change in the time you take it is more likely to result in a pregnancy than if you were taking a combined oral contraceptive. The POP absolutely needs to be taken at the same time every day. Its greatest effect on the cervical mucus peaks within 2-3 hours after the pill has been taken and then gradually diminishes. After 24 hours the cervical mucus has returned to almost normal. To get the greatest protection, it is best to set up your POP schedule so you take a pill a few hours before you are most likely to have intercourse *(not right before)*, and then stick to that regimen. Some women find it easy to remember to take a POP because it is a daily event.

Minipill effectiveness may also depend on the dose, since the amount of the progestin in the available brands may not be enough for some women, particularly very large women. In several studies, pregnancies occurred most often among women who weighed over 155 pounds.

NOTE: Like combined oral contraceptives, progestin-only pills do not offer any protection against AIDS and other sexually transmitted diseases. Male condoms with spermicide offer the best protection against bacteria and viruses. Abstinence or a long-term, mutually faithful relationship are the only other truly effective ways to protect yourself.

IN A NUTSHELL

POPs

Progestin-only pills (POPs) are birth control pills that contain only one hormone, a progestin, instead of two. They are not as likely to cause side effects such as nausea or breast tenderness. Women who take them may also have less risk of serious side effects like blood clots and strokes. POPs also can be taken by women who are breastfeeding.

POPs are likely to cause changes in your periods. You may have irregular periods, light periods, or none at all.

Because this type of Pill has only one hormone, it must be taken at exactly the same time every day. ANY CHANGE in the time you take this pill will reduce its protection. If you have a hard time sticking to a strict schedule, POPs may not be the right birth control for you.

To get a prescription for progestin-only pills, you must be examined by your doctor or nurse. There are only three brands of POPs. Not all drugstores sell all three, but most will order them for you.

Progestin-only birth control pills do not protect you against any STDs, including AIDS.

Reversibility

Women who stop using the POP appear to return to their normal fertility much more quickly than women who use the combination pills. When a woman has difficulty conceiving after going off POPs, the reasons often are her age, a physical condition that existed before she started the pill, or an unrelated condition that developed during the time she was taking it.

HEALTH EFFECTS

Because so few women use progestin-only pills, there have not been any large studies to demonstrate particular health benefits or disadvantages. They are thought to be safer, at least in theory, than estrogen-containing oral contraceptives, while providing many of the same benefits.

Advantages of POPs

Because they contain no estrogen, progestin-only pills cause fewer serious complications and side effects than combined oral contraceptives. If you have a cardiovascular health problem that does not allow you to use a combined oral contraceptive, you may do well on POPs. If you developed high blood pressure or headaches while taking the combined pill, POPs may be a better oral contraceptive for you.

Minipills have not been found to increase the risk of cancers, and they are less likely to cause some of the side effects seen with combined pills, such as depression, nausea, breast tenderness, acne, and unwanted hair growth. They may be a good choice if you are diabetic. The minipill is also useful if you want to breastfeed and to use an oral contraceptive. It is best, however, to start using POPs after breastfeeding is well established. (See Chapter 17 for information on breastfeeding and contraceptive use.)

Most of the health benefits of progestin-only pills are similar to those of combined oral contraceptives: a decrease in menstrual cramps or pain, less heavy bleeding, and a lessening of premenstrual syndrome (PMS) symptoms.

Possible Risks of the Minipill

Functional Ovarian Cysts. As we explained in Chapter 7, during the menstrual cycle some follicles in the ovaries do not rupture or disappear as they normally would, but enlarge and become cysts instead. Although these cysts rarely produce symptoms, some may cause pelvic pain, pain during intercourse, or unusually heavy or painful periods. Women using progestin-only pills are at a slightly greater than average risk of developing this problem. If the cysts cause symptoms, your health care provider may recommend that you use another contraceptive method. Most cysts disappear in a few months without treatment.

Ectopic Pregnancy. If pregnancy does occur when you are using the minipill, your risk of having an ectopic (tubal) pregnancy is somewhat higher than usual. A possible explanation is that the minipill does not always stop ovulation, but can slow the transport of the egg through the fallopian tubes. Symptoms of an ectopic pregnancy include sudden abdominal pain and unexpected vaginal spotting or bleeding.

Breast Cancer. There appears to be no greater risk of breast cancer among women who use progestin-only contraceptives. If you already have breast cancer, however, you should not use any oral contraceptive.

Common Complaints or Side Effects

Menstrual Disturbances. Expect to experience changes in your menstrual periods when you start taking the minipill. If ovulation stops, you will be completely protected against pregnancy and you probably will have very irregular periods or none at all. If you continue to have regular periods, you are probably still ovulating, at least some of the time. You will need to be careful in your use of the POP and in using backup contraception if you miss a pill or take one late.

Erratic bleeding patterns are the most notable side effect, common to all progestin-only methods, including the minipill. It is not unusual to have periods of light bleeding that last longer or are spaced closer together. Sometimes menstrual periods are fairly regular, but there is breakthrough bleeding between them. Shortened cycles are common. Long episodes of bleeding or no bleeding at all happen less often. Many women will have less bleeding overall, which means they are less likely to be anemic.

Although menstruation that is unpredictable or more frequent is annoying, it is not a health problem. The frequency of short cycles seems to decrease with time. If you continue to find your menstrual changes annoying, talk to your health care provider about switching methods.

However, if you stop having periods after you have already been on the minipill for some time, it could be an indication of pregnancy, and you should talk immediately to your health care provider about a pregnancy test. Also consult your provider if you experience prolonged episodes of bleeding or have severe abdominal pain.

Cautions

Effect on the Fetus. If you take oral contraceptives after you unknowingly have become pregnant, the risk of your child having any abnormality will not increase above the usual 5 to 6 percent risk that exists for all pregnancies.

Drug Interactions. POPs can be made less effective by some commonly prescribed drugs that speed up liver activity, which may lead to breakthrough bleeding or even pregnancy, although this occurs rarely. Drugs that may affect the performance of the minipill include prescription headache pills containing barbiturates such as butalbital (Fiorinal, Fioricet, Esgic), the tuberculosis antibiotic rifampin, the oral antifungal drug griseofulvin (Fulvicin, Grifulvin, Grisactin), and antiseizure drugs containing carbamazepine (Tegretol), phenytoin (Dilantin), primidone (Mysoline), or phenobarbital. If you take such medications regularly, progestin-only pills are not recommended. New antiseizure drugs like Neurontin and Lamictal may be less likely to interact with birth control pills.

Whenever a drug is prescribed for you, remind your medical provider of the other medications you are using. It is a good idea to remind your pharmacist also.

Breastfeeding. Unlike contraceptives that contain estrogen, progestin-only pills do not reduce the amount of breast milk. A small amount of the hormone does get into breast milk, however, although this has not been found to have a negative effect on babies. If you strongly prefer birth control pills over other methods of contraception, the progestin-only pill is the best choice while you nurse your baby.

If you do not breastfeed or if you nurse but also give your baby supplementary foods, you should begin taking the minipill soon after delivery, because you will begin ovulating again. For convenience, you may want to ask your health care provider for a POP prescription before the birth or soon after. When you stop breastfeeding, you can either continue with the progestin-only pill or you can switch to the combined pill. Breastfeeding women who are fully nursing and whose periods have not started can delay the use of other contraceptive methods for a while. Information on breastfeeding and contraception is given in Chapter 17.

HOW TO USE THE PROGESTIN-ONLY PILL

To determine if a you are a good candidate for the minipill, a personal and family health history is taken by a health care provider. A physical examination, including a pelvic exam and a Pap test, is also necessary.

If you are under age 18 and wonder if the clinic or physician will tell your parents about your visit, you may find it helpful to ask some of the privacy questions listed on page 234 in Chapter 18.

Progestin-only pills rely on a very low dose of a single hormone. To maintain their impact on the cervical mucus, POPs must be taken every day, at the same time each day. This is unlike combined oral contraceptives, most of which have a 7-day drug-free interval. (Some versions of the Pill are taken every day but the last week of pills are nonactive.) The effects of the minipill last for barely 24 hours before they wear off. As we noted, the greatest impact on the cervical mucus is achieved within 2 to 3 hours after you have swallowed the pill.

The kinds of errors that threaten the minipill's effectiveness include: (1) taking a pill more than 3 hours late, (2) forgetting to take a pill for 1 day or more, and (3) not using a backup method when a pill is taken late, missed, vomited up, or taken with medicine that weakens its potency.

Start the pill on the first day of your period. Take one pill each day until you have finished the packet; then start a new packet the very next day. With the minipill you must never skip a day. Your pharmacy will probably let you buy two packets at the beginning, or you can ask your doctor to write the prescription for two packets rather than one. When you finish the first pack, buy another. This way you will always have a package of pills in reserve.

Use a backup method of birth control for the first 7 days. It will take at least a week for the pill to achieve its several effects during your first cycle. To be extra safe, you may want to use your backup for the first month, to make sure you can stick to the rigid schedule the minipill method requires. Condoms, foam, a diaphragm with a spermicide, or contraceptive film are good backup choices. No methods that rely on body temperature or mucus quality (natural methods) should be used at the same time as POPs, since the hormone in the pill will change all these natural signals. Always keep a backup contraceptive handy in case you forget to refill your prescription or must discontinue POPs for some reason.

Link your pill-taking with another daily activity. Make it easy to follow your pill schedule. Women who usually have intercourse at night should schedule their pill-taking with dinner. And, if you take your pill in the evening, you will still be protected the next morning or afternoon. The fact that you must take the pill at the same time every day does not mean you can have sex only at set times. But it does make sense to be most protected when you most likely will have intercourse.

Vomiting or severe diarrhea. Your intestinal system may not absorb the progestin if you are having severe diarrhea or vomiting. If you vomit within 2 hours after taking a minipill, take another one and stay with your pill regimen. Use your backup contraceptive if you have sex while you are sick and for at least 7 days afterwards.

If you miss one minipill. If you miss taking a pill, take the pill you missed as soon as you remember. Also take the next pill at the regular time even if it means taking two pills in one day. If you are more than 3 hours late taking the minipill, also use your backup method for 7 days when you have sex.

If you miss two or more minipills in a row. Miss taking two or more pills in a row, and you could become pregnant. Start using your backup method right away. Take two pills every day until you have used up the pills you have missed. Continue to use your backup method for 7 days beyond the day your pill-taking went back on schedule.

Lighter and shorter periods. You may bleed for only a couple of days, or only have some spotting. The blood may be brownish in

ARE YOU A GOOD CANDIDATE FOR POPs?

If you tend to be disorganized or forgetful or if your daily routine is unpredictable, you may find that the rigid pill-taking schedule necessary with the progestin-only pill may not work for you. There is very little margin of error with this method. Even a minor delay in pill-taking can make you susceptible to pregnancy.

If you are breastfeeding or over age 35, it is likely that your fertility is diminished. The minipill can be a good choice for you—if your lifestyle allows you stick to a schedule.

color. Your periods may become shorter or very irregular. For example, you may have a 28-day cycle, followed by a 17-day cycle, followed by a 35-day cycle. Some of these irregularities may correct themselves after a few months; some may not. None of these changes is medically important.

Breakthrough bleeding. If you have breakthrough spotting or bleeding between your menstrual periods, continue to take your pills on schedule. In most cases, bleeding between periods stops in a few days. Breakthrough bleeding is not unusual during the first few months of taking the minipill. It may occur if you have missed one or more pills. If it continues beyond the first 4 or 5 months, see your health care practitioner.

Heavy bleeding and cramps. If the bleeding is uncommonly heavy for you, or if you have unusual cramps, pain, or fever, see your practitioner. These can be signs of an ectopic pregnancy or infection.

If your period is overdue but you have not forgotten any pills, it does not mean you are pregnant. It is not remarkable to miss a period occasionally while taking progestin-only pills. If you are worried about being pregnant, contact your health care provider.

If you miss a period and have forgotten one or more minipills during that cycle, particularly early in the cycle, there is a chance that you are pregnant. Contact your clinic or doctor for an early pregnancy test. A blood pregnancy test (one that uses a blood sample) can be accurate approximately 1 week after conception. A urine pregnancy test is accurate 10 to 14 days after the missed period, or about 4 weeks after conception. Home pregnancy tests are accurate only if the directions on the package are followed carefully. If used too early, they may give a false negative result.

Keep a record of your periods. If 45 days have passed since the beginning of your last menstrual period and you suspect you may be pregnant, call your doctor or clinic to arrange for an early pregnancy test. This is especially important if you have been sick or have missed more than one pill without using your backup method of birth control.

If your pregnancy test is negative, discuss with your health care provider whether you should have a second test, especially if you have symptoms like morning sickness or enlarged breasts that are signs of pregnancy.

COST

The expense of using any oral contraceptive, including the minipill, includes a physical examination and perhaps laboratory tests. Physicals can range in cost from $60 to $175, plus charges for the tests. The amount depends on whether you go to a private physician or health care center, a government-funded clinic, or to Planned Parenthood or another nonprofit women's health care center. Some government-funded clinics charge a sliding fee, which generally means you pay according to your income. If you belong to an HMO, the cost is the usual modest co-payment for the physical and for filling the prescription every month. Some, but not many, commercial insurance plans also cover the expense of minipill prescriptions—check your plan.

The price of minipills ranges from $26 to just over $30 for a month's supply, depending on the pharmacy filling the prescription. Not all drugstores carry all three brands of minipills, although they

PROGESTIN-ONLY PILLS

Product	Dose	Manufacturer
Micronor	28-day pack or dispenser	Ortho
Nor-QD	42-tablet pack	Roche
Ovrette	6 dispensers/28 tablets each	Wyeth-Ayerst

are usually willing to order them. Because even a modest variation in cost adds up over the months, it is worth shopping around for the lowest price. As usual, minipills cost less at women's health centers, Planned Parenthood, public clinics, and large chain drugstores.

9

Norplant

Norplant consists of six flexible, slender capsules that are inserted just under the skin on the inside of the upper arm. They can be felt by the fingers and sometimes their outline may be visible. Norplant delivers levonorgestrel, a progestin commonly used in contraceptive pills, via a system that was invented more than 25 years ago. The porous, silicone capsules allow the levonorgestrel to enter the bloodstream slowly, providing the body with a continuous low dose of progestin day after day. This results in hormone levels that are lower than those from a daily minipill. Because Norplant is a hormone method, it has some of the same side effects as birth control pills. It also may cause bleeding disturbances—at least for the first months of use.

Norplant is effective for 5 years. The capsules then must be removed and replaced, if desired, by a new set.

The main advantages of Norplant are: (1) There is nothing to take and no prescription to refill every month. (2) It is almost as effective as sterilization, yet the contraceptive effect disappears soon after the capsules are removed. (3) A pelvic examination is not necessary with Norplant, although it is recommended. (4) Except in women with thin arms, the capsules are not visible, so only you

IN A NUTSHELL

NORPLANT

Norplant is a birth control method that uses six tiny capsules that contain a progestin. They are placed just under the skin on the inside of the upper arm. In most women they are barely visible.

The capsules are porous, which means they allow small, regular amounts of progestin to pass into the body and prevent pregnancy. They hold enough progestin to last for 5 years.

Before the capsules are inserted, the skin is made numb in that part of your arm. Then the capsules are inserted with an instrument like a fat ballpoint pen.

The most common side effect is irregular bleeding. This irregularity varies from woman to woman. Some have prolonged menstrual bleeding during the first months afterwards or untimely bleeding or spotting between periods, no bleeding at all, or a combination of these.

With Norplant, there is nothing to remember and no prescription to refill every month. It is extremely effective, yet after it is removed, your periods start again and you can get pregnant almost right away.

Although having Norplant inserted is expensive, it costs less than 5 years of most other types of contraceptives.

Norplant does not protect you against STDs, including AIDS.

know you are using a contraceptive. (5) Although the up-front cost is high, when compared to the expense of 5 years of other methods, it is much cheaper than most.

Norplant's greatest disadvantage is that having it inserted and removed is expensive. In addition, the removal procedure can be uncomfortable, and the bleeding irregularities can be annoying to some women.

When Norplant is inserted, there is an initial surge of hormone that gradually diminishes until the capsules are delivering only a little bit of progestin every day. This means that only a tiny amount of hormone is necessary to produce a good contraceptive effect. The low dose of progestin and the absence of estrogen make Norplant a very safe contraceptive method.

Like the minipill, the progestin in Norplant prevents pregnancy by thickening the cervical mucus so it is difficult for sperm to penetrate. It also inhibits ovulation so eggs are not produced regularly, and it makes the womb inhospitable to a fertilized egg.

The Norplant tubes are made of the same silicone used for other medical devices such as some heart valves. Tubing made of this material has been used safely in surgical procedures since the 1950s. The Norplant capsules are tiny and contain 100 times less silicone than do silicone gel breast implants.

The six capsules are placed under the skin through a single small puncture-type incision that is about 1/8 inch wide, using an instrument that resembles a fat ballpoint pen with a sharp tip (Figure 9.1). The procedure generally takes 10 to 20 minutes and is done with a local anesthetic injected near the area. No stitches are required. If you are right-handed, the capsules are inserted in the left arm; if you are left-handed, the right arm is used. A health care provider who inserts Norplant should be specially trained before he or she performs this procedure.

The capsules can be removed at any time; fertility returns almost immediately afterwards. At the end of the fifth year, the method begins to become less effective, so if you want to continue with it, the old capsules must be replaced with new ones.

This system of long-lasting hormonal implants has been used in

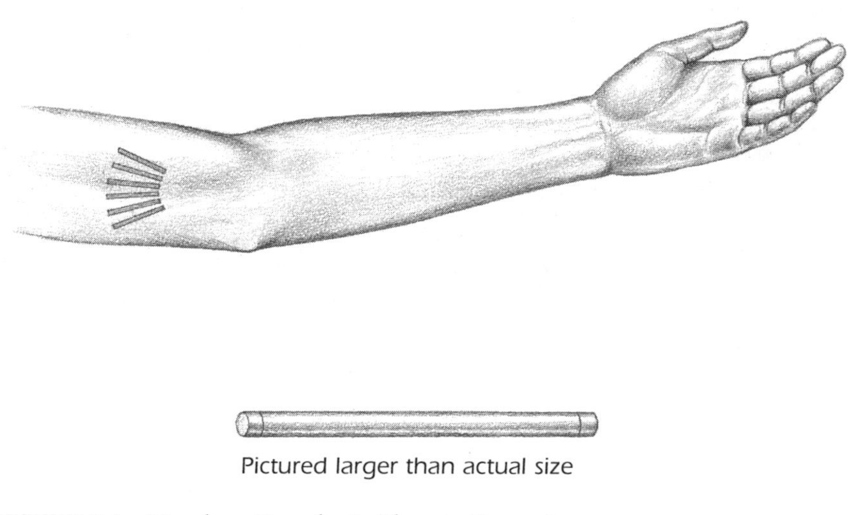

FIGURE 9.1 Norplant Capsules in Place in Upper Arm.

other countries since 1983, and was approved in the U.S. in late 1990. More than three million women around the world have now used Norplant. Women like this method because they do not have to remember to take a pill every day or interrupt their lovemaking to insert something.

Norplant does not protect against sexually transmitted diseases.

EFFECTIVENESS AND REVERSIBILITY

Norplant is a highly reliable form of birth control, because there are no pills to forget or prescription to renew. Yet normal fertility returns very soon after the capsules have been removed.

Failure Rate

Although its hormone dose is extremely small, the failure rate for Norplant during the first 12 months after insertion is just under 1 percent. Over a 5-year period of use the failure rate is a bit more than 1 percent.

The implants begin releasing hormone directly into the bloodstream immediately after insertion. If you get the implants during the first 7 days of your menstrual cycle, no backup method is needed. If the insertion takes place at any other time during your monthly cycle, you will need backup contraception during the first 24 hours.

Reversibility

When the Norplant capsules are removed, it is possible to conceive quite soon, so you must start on another method of birth control the same day if you do not want to get pregnant. This is in contrast to women who discontinue oral contraceptives containing estrogen and progestin, who sometimes find that several months or more may elapse before they are ovulating regularly again and are able to conceive.

NORPLANT AND SILICONE

The silicone in Norplant has been used for many years in a variety of medical replacements for body parts. Recent studies involving thousands of patients have not found that silicone increases the risk of autoimmune disorders. The most recent study on thousands of women with breast implants was published in the New England Journal of Medicine in June, 1994.

Before these studies, a huge class-action lawsuit against the maker of silicone breast implants was won. Because of its success, lawyers began to advertise for clients who ever received a medical device containing silicone or had a problem with Norplant. Some lawyers are irresponsibly telling women who have had no problems with Norplant to have their implants removed and to sue the manufacturer.

It is hoped that the current false alarms being raised by lawyers who are seeking financial gain will not frighten women away from a very effective contraceptive.

HEALTH EFFECTS

Health effects of Norplant may include:

Irregular Bleeding. The most common side effect of progestin-only contraceptives is a change in menstrual bleeding, such as heavy or irregular bleeding, spotting between periods, prolonged episodes of bleeding and spotting, or no bleeding at all. Although a period may last for more days than usual, the total blood loss is usually less than before. With Norplant, amenorrhea (no monthly periods) is most likely to occur during the first year of use, because progestin amounts are slightly higher then. Menstrual periods sometimes return in the second year as the daily progestin amount drops a little. If the irregularity in your periods bothers you a lot, you may want to switch to another method.

Headaches. Some women experience an increase in the number or severity of headaches. Some may start having migraines. Usually this reaction disappears after a few months, but if it does not, it may be necessary to remove the implant.

Breast Tenderness. This occurs in a few women and occasionally can be very painful. Although pregnancy is unlikely, a pregnancy test should be done, just to be sure.

Mood Changes and Depression. If depression, anxiety, and other mood changes persist beyond the first months and are severe, removing the implant may be necessary.

Drug Interactions. Like progestin-only pills, Norplant can be made less effective by some commonly prescribed drugs that speed up liver activity, which may lead to breakthrough bleeding or even pregnancy. Drugs that may affect Norplant's performance include prescription headache pills which contain barbiturates (Fiorinal, Fioricet, Esgic), the tuberculosis antibiotic rifampin, the oral antifungal drug griseofulvin (Fulvicin, Grifulvin, Grisactin), and the antiseizure drugs containing carbamazepine (Tegretol), phenytoin (Dilantin), primidone (Mysoline), or phenobarbital. If you take such medications regularly, Norplant may not be recommended. The possibility of a drug interaction should be discussed with your physician. There are too few women taking these drugs while using Norplant to study for definite answers. If you already are using Norplant and must take such medications, you may want to add the extra protection of a condom or spermicide.

When you are using a hormonal method, you should always remind your health care provider of this fact when discussing any prescription.

Ovarian Cysts. Functional ovarian cysts (enlarged follicles) are uncommon but sometimes occur in Norplant users just as they may occur in women who do not use Norplant. They may produce some discomfort, but usually disappear on their own. If you should experience severe abdominal pain or unusually heavy or painful periods, however, get in touch with your physician.

Inflammation or Infection at the Insertion Site. These complications can occur after any minor or major surgical procedure. Any pus or bleeding at the insertion site should be brought to the attention of your health care provider.

Acne. Acne is the most common skin reaction in Norplant users. If you are particularly concerned about this possibility, ask your health care provider to prescribe the progestin-only pill Ovrette so you can see what happens to your skin under the influence of levonorgestrel. If Ovrette gives you acne, so will Norplant. However, there are a number of prescription medications that treat acne successfully.

Other Side Effects. Other, less common side effects include unwanted hair growth, nervousness, nausea, dizziness, change in appetite, and hair loss. These reactions may disappear after several months or become much less noticeable. Many women report a small weight gain when using Norplant, but usually less than with an injectable contraceptive.

IS NORPLANT RIGHT FOR YOU?

This method of birth control is especially appealing to some women because it provides continuous protection against pregnancy for 5 years without any special effort.

Good Candidates

All women. Norplant is suitable for almost all women who are seeking continuous, highly effective yet reversible, contraception. Progestin implants are particularly appropriate for women who cannot use methods that contain estrogen. For women of all ages, Norplant is desirable because they do not have to remember to take a pill every day or to renew their prescriptions. When a pregnancy is wanted, Norplant is easily reversible. An older woman can use Norplant comfortably as she approaches menopause.

Breastfeeding women. Like all hormonal contraceptives, Norplant is not the first choice for the breastfeeding woman, but if she prefers to use a hormonal method, she should choose one with no estrogen, such as Norplant. (For more information on breastfeeding and birth control, see Chapter 17.)

Women with diabetes or a history of heart disease. Women with these problems should not use a birth control method that contains estrogen, so Norplant is a good choice, because it is a progestin-only method.

Women Who Are Not Good Candidates

Women who have active thromboembolic disorders, such as blood clots in their legs, lungs, or eyes. Women who have had these problems should talk to their health care providers about whether to use Norplant.

Women with unexplained vaginal bleeding. The irregular bleeding that goes along with Norplant may obscure any unusual bleeding that can be a symptom of cancer of the reproductive tract. If a woman already has unusual bleeding, she should not start on Norplant until the explanation for that bleeding has been found.

Women with acute liver disease, or liver tumors. The hormones are metabolized by the liver so you need a good, working liver to handle this drug.

Women who smoke. Smoking greatly increases the probability of a heart attack or stroke for anyone. This risk is strongly aggravated by the use of combined (estrogen-progestin) oral contraceptives. While this is believed to be an estrogen-related effect, it also may be linked to the progestin. Even though Norplant does not contain estrogen, a woman who chooses to use it is advised not to smoke.

Women who cannot tolerate irregular bleeding. If having regular periods is important to you, Norplant and other progestin-only methods are not good choices.

CHOOSING NORPLANT

Because Norplant requires minor surgery for insertion and removal, you will want to learn as much as you can about this method before you use it.

Finding a Practitioner

Although the procedure for inserting Norplant capsules is very simple, it is important that it be performed correctly. If the capsules are inserted too deeply, they are more difficult to remove later. The U.S. distributor of Norplant, Wyeth-Ayerst Laboratories, has trained over 25,000 health care providers to insert the capsules. These include doctors, nurse-midwives, nurse-practitioners, and other medical professionals. You should be able to find a practitioner who has been trained in the technique by calling Wyeth's Norplant hotline: 1-800-934-5556. Your local Planned Parenthood affiliate, a nearby woman's health clinic, or the obstetrics/gynecology service of your local hospital may also provide Norplant.

When asking about a practitioner, be sure you are clear about wanting someone who has been trained and has had experience in inserting the capsules. The more often providers perform this procedure, the more skilled they become, and this means a faster, more comfortable experience for you. And the capsules will be placed exactly where they should be.

If you are concerned about the privacy of any birth control method you might use, you should be aware that the Norplant capsules can be felt and sometimes can be seen under the skin of your upper arm.

Norplant Counseling

If you have doubts about any aspects of Norplant, do not hesitate to ask questions. Before your appointment, write down any anxieties you have so you do not forget to have them resolved. Do not be reluctant to ask how often the practitioner has inserted

Norplant capsules. There is nothing wrong with being nervous about the insertion procedure or about the possible side effects this method could have. It is only sensible to clear up any questions you have about Norplant before the capsules have been inserted, no matter how "dumb" you think your questions are. A good health care provider will not mind answering questions.

The more you know about Norplant and its effects beforehand, the more at ease you will be with any reaction you experience. You should not be reluctant to contact your practitioner afterward, especially about changes in your body or menstrual pattern, if you are not entirely comfortable with them. *Do not have the implants inserted until you are sure you understand what the side effects of this method are and exactly what happens during the procedure.*

The Procedure

To avoid the risk of placing the capsules in a woman who is pregnant, providers are advised to implant the capsules during the first 7 days of the menstrual cycle or immediately after an abortion.

The site usually selected for the implants is on the inner side of the arm, a few inches above the bend of the elbow. If there is some reason this is not a good place for you, discuss this with the practitioner. Most practitioners will draw a mark on your arm showing where the capsules will be placed in a fan-shaped pattern. A local anesthetic is injected before the capsule insertion and the injection may sting for a second or two. After the area is numb, a tiny incision is made and, using a special needle, the capsules are placed one at a time under the skin so they do not touch each other and the progestin can diffuse easily from each one.

The insertion process takes 10 to 20 minutes. There are no stitches. After the anesthetic wears off, the insertion area will feel sore and may be bruised and swollen for a few days. Some women feel a little tingling or numbness afterwards.

The incision is covered by a small gauze pad and adhesive tape that should be left in place for a few days. Keep that part of your arm dry and protected from dirt until it heals. Try not to bump it and do not lift anything heavy for several days.

Because the incision is so tiny, it seldom leaves a detectable scar. The implants are comfortable and barely visible. Although you may be aware of them, almost no one else will notice their existence.

The capsules do not move around and, because they are flexible, they cannot break, no matter how vigorously you use your arm. After the incision is healed, you can treat that arm as you normally would. You can put pressure on the area or touch the skin without concern. You can swim, play sports, carry packages, and do heavy work.

LIVING WITH NORPLANT

Warning Signs of Possible Problems

Serious problems are rare, but you should call your health care provider immediately if you develop severe lower abdominal pain, heavy vaginal bleeding, migraine or other severe headaches, visual disturbances, or if a capsule works its way out through the skin. It is unusual for a capsule to come out spontaneously. If it does, it may be the result of being inserted not quite deep enough or because of an infection at the site. Call your health care provider.

Pain in the implant arm, or pus or bleeding at the site of the implant may indicate an infection, and you should see your provider right away.

You should also check with your physician or nurse if you have a delayed period after a number of regular menstrual cycles, because this could be a sign of pregnancy.

Dealing with Menstrual Irregularity

Irregular or heavy menstrual periods, spotting between periods, or no periods at all are common among users of progestin implants, especially during the first year. There is no harm if you do not menstruate; the blood does not accumulate in your uterus. What happens is that the lining of the uterus does not thicken and become filled with blood every month as it otherwise would, so there is little or no blood to be shed. The absence of menstrual periods does not mean you are pregnant, nor does it mean you will have problems becoming pregnant after your implants are removed. If you are worried that you might be pregnant, take a pregnancy test to put your mind at rest. If your periods do not return after a year, you probably will have few, if any, bleeding days each month while you are using Norplant.

If such menstrual irregularity bothers you, talk to your health care practitioner. Most bleeding irregularities associated with Norplant use are not serious, although in rare cases persistent spotting could be an indication of a cervical infection or malignancy. Spotting does not mean you cannot have intercourse and it does not make you anemic. Although the spotting may be continuous, you are probably losing less, rather than more, blood than usual. Prolonged, heavy bleeding can result in anemia, however.

Removing and Replacing Capsules

When you have Norplant inserted, your practitioner will probably give you a booklet for writing down the date the capsules were inserted, by whom and where, and when they should be removed. You should store this somewhere for future reference. If you keep a calendar, you can record this information and then carry it forward to your new calendar every year so you know when you must have your implants removed.

Norplant capsules should be removed after 5 years because after this time they gradually become less effective. They also can be taken out at any earlier time and for any reason.

As with the insertion, you should make sure that the nurse or doctor who will be doing the removal has been trained to perform the procedure.

Removal can be more difficult than the insertion. The incision for removal may need to be a bit longer than the original. A local anesthetic is injected at the end of the capsules. If you still feel some pain, tell your practitioner so you can be given extra anesthetic. Because they are visible with either x-rays or ultrasound, Norplant capsules are easily located. On rare occasions, a second visit is needed to get out all the capsules.

After the removal procedure, you will have some swelling and bruising similar to the aftereffects of the insertion. These will wear off in a few days. If your arm is very uncomfortable, ask your provider about taking something to ease the pain.

As soon as the capsules are removed, you will need to have another set inserted or start using another method if you want to avoid pregnancy.

COST

The Norplant implant alone costs $365. The practitioner's fee for the insertion procedure is additional and will vary, depending on whether it is done by a private physician or in a publicly funded clinic, and can range from $50 to $400. If you keep your capsules for the full 5 years, the cost averages out to approximately $80 to $150 a year.

Most or all of the cost of a Norplant insertion—the implant plus the insertion—is covered by Medicaid in many states, as well as by some health insurance plans. HMOs charge their usual modest co-payment for the exam and insertion.

If the removal procedure is not covered by insurance, low-income women may be able to obtain funding through the Norplant Foundation. For more information about financial help for removing Norplant, call 1-800-760-9030.

10

Depo-Provera

Depo-Provera is another progestin-only birth control method. It is an injection that protects against pregnancy for 3 months. Although Depo-Provera has been available for years in over 90 other countries and has been used by millions of women, it did not receive FDA approval in the United States until 1992. Since then it has become an extremely popular contraceptive, and at some women's clinics it rivals the Pill in the number of women using it.

The progestin used in the injection, Depo-medroxyprogesterone acetate (DMPA), inhibits ovulation by suppressing the amounts of luteinizing hormone and follicle-stimulating hormone that a woman's body usually produces in order to ovulate. Like other progestins, DMPA also makes the uterus inhospitable to any possible fertilized egg, and thickens the cervical mucus so it discourages the passage of sperm.

After the injection, the DMPA acts like a timed-release "depot" of progestin in the muscle. Low levels are released constantly into the circulation until the depot is exhausted.

Depo-Provera injections are given once every 3 months to maintain contraceptive impact and are more than 99 percent effective. Studies thus far show no serious side effects from the use of DMPA.

Like the other progestin-only methods, however, Depo-Provera generally causes many months of irregular bleeding, usually followed by no bleeding at all.

Like all hormonal methods, injections of DMPA do not protect against AIDS or other sexually transmitted diseases.

EFFECTIVENESS AND REVERSIBILITY

Depo-Provera is highly effective as long as you are consistent in returning to the clinic for your next shot. When it is discontinued, however, normal fertility may not return as readily for some women as it does when other progestin-only methods are stopped.

Failure Rate

The failure rate for Depo-Provera is less than 1 percent. The injection (150 mg) is designed to last a little longer than 3 months, just in case it is not possible to return to the clinic or physician's office exactly on schedule.

Reversibility

The effects of Depo-Provera do not disappear as rapidly as the other progestin-only methods, and a number of months may pass after the last injection before fertility is restored. Studies found that 68 percent of the women who did become pregnant after discontinuing Depo-Provera did so within 12 months. Almost all women conceived within 18 months after the last injection. Women with lower body weights became pregnant sooner than women with higher body weights. The length of time it took to become pregnant was not related to the duration of Depo-Provera use.

This long-lasting effect does not apply to all women, however. If you give up this method but do not wish to become pregnant, to be safe you must start using another contraceptive method within three months after your final Depo-Provera injection.

IN A NUTSHELL

DEPO-PROVERA

Depo-Provera is a progestin that is given as an injection every 3 months to prevent pregnancy. It is very effective and easy to use because you do not have to remember to take a pill every day or get a prescription refilled.

Depo-Provera does not protect you against STDs. For protection against diseases, you or your partner need to use a condom as well.

To have regular Depo-Provera shots, you need to go to a clinic like Planned Parenthood or to a doctor.

The most common side effect is a change in your periods. Eventually some women have no periods at all. If you stop having the injections, your periods will start again.

HEALTH EFFECTS

Irregular Bleeding. Like other progestin-only contraceptives, Depo-Provera changes your menstrual cycle. It produces irregular periods, long periods of light bleeding or spotting, or no periods at all (amenorrhea). Some women have more days of heavy bleeding, although the total amount of blood they lose is not increased. Irregular bleeding patterns can be annoying, but they decrease with time and eventually, for most women, menstruation stops. If you can wait, you eventually will have no periods at all, which many women find is a comfortable state of affairs. Depo-Provera suppresses the hormones that usually activate the ovaries. Over a period of time, this causes the ovaries to rest and not produce eggs. The regular monthly enrichment of the endometrium does not take place, so there is little or no menstruation. If Depo-Provera is stopped, menstrual periods gradually return to normal.

Weight Gain and Bloating. It is not unusual to gain a few pounds while using Depo-Provera, and some women gain so much weight they change to another method of birth control. Fluid retention also may occur. If you have epilepsy, asthma, or migraine headaches, and you experience bloating, bring this reaction to the attention of your physician.

Headaches. Some women will experience an increase in the number or intensity of headaches. If this reaction does not disappear after a few months, it may be necessary to discontinue the injections.

Breast Tenderness. This happens in a few women and sometimes can be very painful. Although pregnancy is unlikely, if breast tenderness appears after you have been on Depo-Provera for some time, you should talk to your health care provider about having a pregnancy test.

Depression. If depression and anxiety occur, especially if you have a history of these problems, use another method.

HDL Changes. Levels of high density lipoprotein (HDL) drop in women using Depo-Provera. If your cholesterol levels are high, your physician should monitor you more frequently while you use this contraceptive method.

Drug Interactions. So far there are no reports of Depo-Provera effectiveness being reduced by the use of antiseizure drugs or the TB antibiotic rifampin. However, Depo-Provera does affect the outcome of some laboratory tests. You should always let your health care providers know you are using hormonal birth control.

Cancers. The progestin in Depo-Provera reduces the risk of endometrial cancer and is expected to reduce the risk of ovarian cancer by suppressing ovulation. It has no effect on breast cancer.

Other Side Effects. Reactions that are less common include dizziness, fatigue, nausea, abdominal pain, backache, hot flashes, leg cramps, and a decreased interest in sex. These may disappear or become much less noticeable after a few months of using the method.

IS DEPO-PROVERA RIGHT FOR YOU?

Good Candidates

All women. Depo-Provera is suitable for almost all women in good health. Because it is a progestin-only contraceptive, it is a particularly good choice for women who cannot or should not take estrogen. This method also is popular because it is an injection given at a clinic, and there is no way to tell that you are using birth control. And it does not interrupt lovemaking.

Breastfeeding women. As with all hormonal methods, Depo-Provera is not the birth control method of first choice for breastfeeding women. If you are breastfeeding and wish to use a hormonal method, however, you should use one that contains only a progestin and no estrogen, such as Depo-Provera. Studies have shown that progestins do not reduce the supply of breast milk. Small amounts of the hormone will be in the breast milk, however, although this has not been shown to have a negative effect on infant growth and development. (For more information on contraception while breastfeeding, see Chapter 17.)

Diabetics. Depo-Provera also is a good method for women with diabetes who do not wish to become pregnant.

Young women and teenagers. Although women of all ages appreciate the advantages of Depo-Provera, it is popular particularly among younger women, because there is little hassle associated with it, no rigid schedule to follow, no prescription that must be refilled and no pills to be remembered. If an appointment is slightly delayed, there is no immediate worry about pregnancy because this method has a 1- to 2-week grace period. Furthermore, the thick cervical mucus that progestin causes seems to offer some protection against pelvic inflammatory disease.

Women with sickle cell anemia or seizures. Both these conditions may be improved by DMPA.

Women who have severe menstrual cramps and other menstrual cycle problems. Progestin-only contraceptives, including Depo-Provera, tend to reduce the intensity of menstrual pain, premenstrual symptoms, heavy bleeding, and midmonth ovulatory pain.

Women Who Are Not Good Candidates

Women with unexplained vaginal bleeding. The unpredictable and irregular bleeding that usually accompanies the first year or so of Depo-Provera may conceal unusual bleeding that can be a symptom of cancer of the reproductive tract. If a woman already has unusual bleeding, Depo-Provera should not be used until the explanation for that bleeding is found.

Women who cannot tolerate irregular bleeding. If having regular periods is important, Depo-Provera and the other progestin-only methods are not good choices.

USING DEPO-PROVERA

After a single 150 mg dose of Depo-Provera is injected, the concentration of the DMPA slowly increases until it reaches a peak level in the bloodstream 3 weeks later. It then very gradually decreases. The DMPA level remains protective against pregnancy for about 13 to 14 weeks. If the time interval between injections is longer than 13 weeks, however, you may need to be tested to make certain you are not pregnant.

Most women's health centers, HMOs, and birth control clinics such as Planned Parenthood offer Depo-Provera as part of their selection of contraceptive methods.

If you are concerned about privacy issues, you may find it helpful to ask the clinic or doctor some of the questions listed on page 234 of Chapter 18.

To begin using this method, you will be asked to call the clinic when your next menstrual period begins. The first Depo-Provera injection is given while you are bleeding to make certain you are not pregnant. If you have just given birth and do not plan to breastfeed, the first injection should be within 5 days of the birth. If you are breastfeeding, the first injection is usually scheduled for the sixth week after the birth. (See Chapter 17 for more information on breastfeeding and contraception.)

Subsequent injections are every 3 months. Clinics use various ways to remind their clients about the next shot. Some simply give you a calendar on which you mark the dates; others will mail you a reminder. If you use a diary or desk calendar, marking it with the day of the next injection is one of the easiest ways to remember.

COST

The costs of the physical examination plus the injection of Depo-Provera vary substantially from area to area. The $120 that Planned Parenthood affiliates and some women's health centers charge for the exam and injection are in the middle of the price range. Subsequent injections commonly are $60 each. The annual expense for four injections is often $240, which compares favorably to the expense of using the Pill. Many HMOs offer Depo-Provera injections and the physical exam for their usual co-payment of $5 to $20. Other health insurance plans and Medicaid often pay for some of the cost of Depo-Provera.

PART THREE

The Intrauterine Method

11

Intrauterine Devices (IUDs)

Intrauterine devices are small and flexible, are made of plastic or plastic and copper, and are placed in the uterus through the cervical opening to prevent conception. An IUD must be put in and removed by a trained health professional. Once the device is in place, a woman is highly protected against pregnancy. Only two types of IUDs are approved by the FDA for use in the United States today: the Progestasert and the ParaGard T380A. The vertical stem of the T-shaped Progestasert contains a modest supply of progesterone that slowly diffuses over a 12-month period, after which this IUD must be removed and replaced. The ParaGard is also T-shaped but is partially copper covered. It is often called the "Copper T." It can be left in place for 10 years.

This form of birth control is extremely effective; it requires almost no attention; and the long-lasting ParaGard is very inexpensive over the long term. It does not interrupt lovemaking, and fertility returns immediately after it has been removed. Furthermore, when an IUD is in place in the uterus, neither partner can feel it. Outside the United States, modern IUDs are the most widely used reversible contraceptives.

The IUD does not protect against sexually transmitted diseases. A woman who has more than one sexual partner or whose partner may have other lovers is at high risk of acquiring STDs and, if she uses an IUD, is more likely to develop pelvic inflammatory disease. To be safe from STDs and PID, it is necessary to use a condom or to be in a long-term, mutually monogamous relationship in which neither partner has an STD.

IUD SAFETY

The IUD was a more common form of contraception in the U.S. during the 1960s and later. Many types were available and one of the most popular was the Dalkon Shield. This all-plastic device had not been reviewed and tested before it was put on the market because, at that time, such devices did not require FDA approval.

The Dalkon Shield was designed with a "tail" composed of "twisted" strings that allowed bacteria to migrate upward into the reproductive organs. This badly designed IUD came on the market during the 1960s. It resulted in so many cases of pelvic inflammatory disease, infected pregnancies, miscarriages, and reproductive system damage—and lawsuits—that the Dalkon Shield was withdrawn from use.

Since then, federal regulations were put in place that require all medical devices, including IUDs, to be tested for safety. To reduce the risk of complications even further, IUD package information was made more explicit and providers became more careful about recommending IUDs.

It is now known that pelvic inflammatory disease can be related to an interaction between the device and the sexual behaviors of the woman and her partner. The device can make it more likely for a local infection to turn into PID. IUDs are not recommended for the woman who changes sexual partners, has had PID since her last pregnancy, or whose partner has other lovers. Some providers do not recommend the IUD to women who may be unusually susceptible to infections because their immune systems are compromised due to AIDS or leukemia.

The Progestasert became available in 1976 and the ParaGard in 1984. A 1989 review of both these IUDs by a diagnostic and therapeutic technology assessment panel found them to be safe and effec-

IN A NUTSHELL

THE IUD

The IUD is a small, T-shaped piece of plastic that is placed in a woman's uterus to prevent pregnancy. One type of IUD is wrapped in copper and can remain in the uterus for as long as 10 years. A second type gives off small amounts of the hormone progesterone for added effectiveness. It must be removed after 1 year.

Not all women can use an IUD. If you have had an infection like gonorrhea, chlamydia, or PID, you may not be able to use the IUD. The IUD is best for women who are in long-term, monogamous relationships.

The IUD does not protect against STDs.

The best time to have an IUD put into your uterus is when you are having your period, so you are sure you are not pregnant. It is also easier to insert it then. This is done during a pelvic examination by a doctor or nurse.

After the IUD is in place, a short string will hang down through the cervix into the back of your vagina. With your finger, you should check for the IUD string once a month. If the string is not there, if you can feel the plastic part of the IUD, or if the device comes out, you must call your clinic right away.

tive. When used by women in mutually faithful relationships, they are extremely reliable in preventing pregnancy and have relatively few complications.

HOW THE IUD WORKS

Any IUD produces a reaction in the uterus that causes the production of white blood cells and substances called prostaglandins. Their presence in the uterus and the fallopian tubes interferes with the movement of sperm and eggs.

If the IUD contains copper, the effect on sperm and eggs is enhanced. Studies among women using copper IUDs have shown very few live sperm in the genital tract, compared to women not using a contraceptive. Copper IUDs exert their contraceptive effects primarily before fertilization—by killing sperm, by impeding the progress of surviving sperm so they fail to reach the fallopian tubes, or by diminishing any survivors' ability to fertilize eggs.

IUDs, particularly copper IUDs, also change egg movement through the fallopian tubes. A comparison of women who used a copper IUD with women who used no contraceptive showed that, after ovulation, none of the eggs from copper IUD users was fertilized, in contrast to more than half the eggs recovered from noncontraceptive users. The eggs were recovered from the fallopian tubes. No eggs were found in the uterus of any of the women using the copper IUD.

TYPES OF IUDs

Two types of IUDs are available in the United States (Figure 11.1). The ParaGard is a copper-covered device that can be left in place for 10 years; the Progestasert is plastic, contains progesterone, and must be replaced after 1 year.

Progestasert

Approved for use in 1976, the Progestasert is a flexible, all plastic, T-shaped IUD with two monofilament (single, nontwisted) threads or strings attached to the base of the vertical stem. The threads hang down into the vagina. They are necessary to indicate that the IUD is in its correct position and are used to remove it. (These threads do not act as a ladder for bacteria.) The arm of the T measures about 1 1/4 inches, and the stem is just under 1 1/2 inches.

The Progestasert continuously emits a small amount of progesterone from its tiny, hollow stem. The hormone provides additional protection against conception. The reservoir releases just slightly more progesterone each day than a woman's body produces in one day during the latter part of a normal menstrual cycle. It acts directly on the lining of the uterus, making it inhospitable to a fertilized egg. Only a tiny amount of progesterone enters the bloodstream, virtually eliminating the side effects that can occur with other progestin methods of birth control. Women who cannot use other hormonal methods for health reasons can use this IUD safely. In addition, the Progestasert reduces menstrual bleeding, which can be a boon for women who have heavy

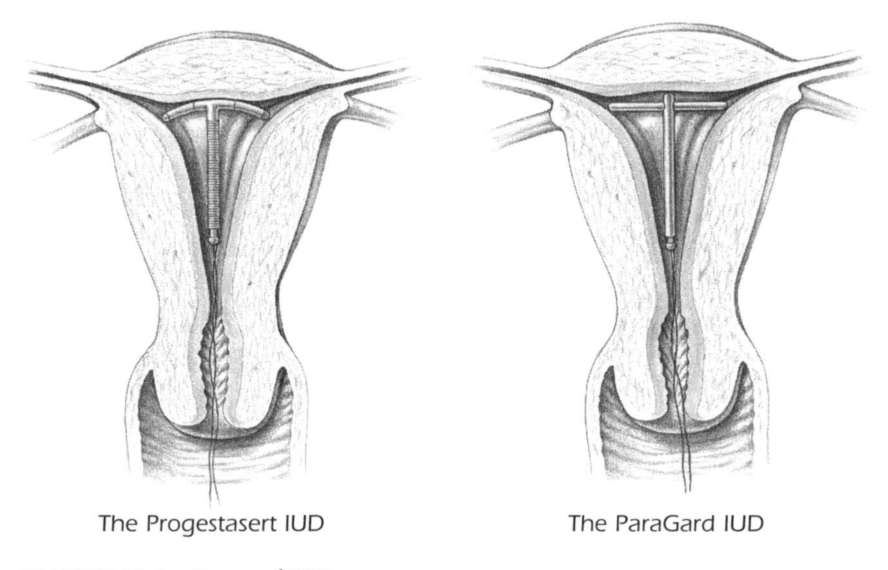

The Progestasert IUD The ParaGard IUD

FIGURE 11.1 Types of IUDs

periods. After 12 months, the supply of the hormone is exhausted, and the Progestasert must be replaced.

The Progestasert is somewhat less effective than the ParaGard and has a slightly higher rate of ectopic pregnancy than the ParaGard or other contraceptives. Furthermore, its short duration of use also presents some disadvantages. Each time an IUD is inserted, there is always a risk that bacteria from the vagina may enter the uterus with it and cause an infection. And there is an expense associated with each insertion and removal.

ParaGard

Copper-covered IUDs have been in use in this country since 1974, ever since researchers found that the addition of copper to the device produced some distinct advantages. More than 20 million have been distributed in over 70 countries. The ParaGard Copper T 380A was approved by the FDA in 1984.

Copper IUDs are less likely to be expelled and do not cause as much menstrual bleeding as did earlier, all-plastic devices. The amount of copper they shed into the body produces no notable side effects. Women allergic to this metal, however, and women with the rare inherited disorder called Wilson's disease, in which excess copper accumulates in body tissues, are advised not to use the ParaGard. The ParaGard is more effective than the Pill and can remain in place for 10 years—a real asset.

The ParaGard is made of polyethylene, with fine copper wire wound around its stem and thin copper "sleeves" on its crosspiece. It is the same size as the Progestasert and also has a pair of monofilament threads extending from the bottom of the stem.

EFFECTIVENESS AND REVERSIBILITY

IUDs are extremely effective and reliable. Normal fertility returns when they are removed.

Failure Rate

Both the Progestasert and the ParaGard have been tested in large clinical trials. The Progestasert has a failure rate of 2 percent or less over a 12-month period; the ParaGard's 12-month failure rate is less than 1 percent.

Reversibility

Fertility returns immediately after an IUD has been removed (or spontaneously expelled).

Good Candidates for this Method

Women who feel they have completed their families and want long-term, highly effective contraception, but are not interested in sterilization, are excellent candidates for an IUD. Because pelvic inflammatory disease is a possible complication with this form of birth control, an IUD is only suitable for the woman who does not have an active or recurrent pelvic infection and is in a long-term,

WHO SHOULD NOT USE AN IUD

You are advised to choose another contraceptive if you have:

- An active or recurrent sexually transmitted disease or other pelvic infection, or a history of STDs or pelvic inflammatory disease. (A yeast infection does not rule out an IUD.)
- More than one sexual partner.
- A sexual partner who has intercourse with others.
- An ectopic pregnancy in the past.
- Undiagnosed, abnormal vaginal bleeding.
- A condition, such as AIDS or leukemia, that may make you more susceptible to infection.
- Wilson's disease or an allergy to copper.

mutually monogamous relationship—so she is not likely to be exposed to a sexually transmitted disease.

CAUTIONS, COMPLICATIONS, AND POSSIBLE SIDE EFFECTS

Cautions

Like most birth control measures, IUDs occasionally can be associated with problems.

Discomfort or pain. If you have never had a child, you are more likely to experience cramps and pain severe enough to need to remove the IUD. Because of the association of IUDs with PID, other methods of contraception preserve fertility better in women who have never had a child and may want one in the future.

Pelvic inflammatory disease. Because an IUD is inserted into the uterus via the vagina and cervical canal, bacteria from those areas can be introduced into the usually sterile uterus, resulting in pelvic inflammatory disease. A vaginal infection should be treated before an IUD is put in. The IUD is not a good choice if you or your partner have a sexually transmitted disease unless you both have been treated successfully for it. IUDs may help STDs ascend into the upper reproductive tract, causing pelvic inflammatory disease.

Undiagnosed abnormal bleeding. The cause of any unusual bleeding should be found before an IUD is used.

Complications

Complications with the IUD can be serious, but they happen only rarely.

Pregnancy. Although pregnancy while using an IUD is uncommon, it may happen, usually because the IUD has unknowingly been expelled or has become embedded in the wall of the uterus. If the woman wishes to continue the pregnancy and the IUD has not been expelled, it should *not* be left in place—if it is, there is more than a 50 percent chance the pregnancy will end in a spontaneous abortion. There also is the possibility of infection. Although these risks are rare, they are real. If the IUD is removed early in the pregnancy, these risks are greatly reduced. If the IUD cannot easily be removed

PELVIC INFLAMMATORY DISEASE (PID)

Women who are not in long-term, mutually faithful relationships today are at risk of having one or more sexually transmitted diseases. If an STD reaches the upper reproductive tract, particularly the fallopian tubes, it can cause pelvic inflammatory disease. PID can damage the fallopian tubes, leading to future ectopic pregnancies and infertility, or to the need for a hysterectomy.

Because many cases of STDs and PID are "silent" and produce no noticeable symptoms, they often are not treated, and the PID can damage fallopian tubes. Severe PID, however, is likely to produce symptoms: chills and fever, abdominal or pelvic pain, an abdomen that is tender to the touch, painful intercourse, severe cramping, and unusual discharge or bleeding. If you develop these symptoms, contact your health care provider at once.

from the uterus, a termination of the pregnancy should be considered. When the IUD is withdrawn and the pregnancy carried full term, no negative effects occur. If you suspect you may be pregnant, get in touch with your health care provider *immediately*.

Ectopic Pregnancy. If you become pregnant while using a Progestasert IUD, the pregnancy is more likely to be ectopic (a tubal pregnancy) than it would be for a woman using another method or the ParaGard. The risk is about the same as it is for a sexually active woman not using birth control.

If you have an ectopic pregnancy, you may develop these symptoms:

- Sudden, severe, or persistent abdominal pain or cramping, often on one side.
- Unusual vaginal bleeding or spotting, along with abdominal pain, especially if this occurs after an unusually light period, or a late or missed period.
- A spell of faintness or dizziness (an indication of internal bleeding), together with any of the preceding symptoms.

You should contact your health care provider at once, because an ectopic pregnancy may rupture at any time. If you cannot reach your doctor, seek help at the nearest hospital emergency room.

Expulsion. Most expulsions take place during the first three months after the IUD has been inserted. The uterus has a natural tendency to expel foreign objects, and the IUD can be pushed out through the cervical opening. It may be expelled by uterine contractions during the first few days of menstruation, when the cervical os is more open. An estimated 2 to 8 percent of IUD users spontaneously expel their IUDs during the first year.

If you find your IUD on a sanitary napkin or in the toilet, obviously it has been expelled. If it has been only partially expelled, you or your partner may feel it in your cervix or vagina. Other signs are pain during intercourse, finding that the IUD threads feel longer, spotting after intercourse or between periods, unusual vaginal discharge, cramps, or pain. If the IUD is expelled without being noticed, the first sign would be missing threads. Pregnancy can occur when the IUD is out of place, so another signal would be signs of pregnancy such as a missed period or morning sickness or tender breasts. It is a good idea to check the threads at least once a month, particularly right after your period.

Perforation. A rare but potentially serious complication of using an IUD is perforation of the uterus (or cervix) by the device. Part of the IUD may penetrate the wall of the uterus or the entire IUD may work its way into the surrounding abdominal cavity. If the IUD traps a loop of the intestine, it could cause a medical emergency. IUDs that perforate the uterus should be removed as soon as the perforation is detected. Removal is usually done via laparoscopy (discussed later in this chapter), but occasionally it can require major surgery. Perforation happens most often at the time the IUD is put in, and it is more likely to occur if the correct technique is not used or if the person doing the insertion it is not thoroughly experienced in the procedure. Perforation is less likely if the health care provider measures the depth and position of the uterus beforehand.

Perforation takes place in approximately one out of every 2,500 insertions. It generally produces no symptoms. The only indication may be the fact you cannot find the threads during your monthly thread-check. Perforations sometimes are discovered only when a woman develops signs of pregnancy. Ultrasound or x-ray can be used to check the position of the IUD.

Embedding. This is a rare and usually less serious complication, in which the lining of the uterus begins to grow around the IUD. An embedded IUD is harder to remove and might break during the removal process. In some cases, a dilatation and curettage (D&C) or other procedure might be necessary to take out the IUD. Threads that seem shorter can be a sign that the IUD is becoming embedded, and this should be brought to the attention of your health care provider right away. Your IUD can be removed and replaced, or you can try another form of birth control.

CHECK YOUR THREADS

Both the ParaGard and the Progestasert have fine polyethylene threads that reach into the vagina so you can feel them with a finger. It is a good idea to check their location before you leave the doctor's office or clinic so you know where they are. Not being able to find them later may mean that the IUD has been expelled or has moved. If this happens, use your backup birth control until the IUD can be checked by your practitioner. You are not protected against pregnancy if your IUD moves out of place.

There are several ways to locate the IUD. Your practitioner can probe the uterus with an instrument or use ultrasound or x-ray to see it. Both the Progestasert and the ParaGard have an opaque material built into them that makes them visible by x-ray. If the IUD is not in the right place, it should be removed. On rare occasions, removal may require surgery.

Infection. Although pelvic infections are not common in healthy women who are not exposed to STDs, there is still some risk. The risk is highest in the months right after an insertion. Since prompt treatment is important, be attentive to possible signs of infection and do not delay seeking treatment if you have: chills and fever, abdominal or pelvic pain, a tender abdomen, severe cramping, painful sex, or any unusual vaginal bleeding or discharge. Even if you are not sure it is a symptom, check with your health care provider.

Side Effects

Bleeding. The most common adverse effects you might experience while using the ParaGard IUD are spotting between periods, or longer and sometimes heavier periods. These problems often diminish over the first few months. Sometimes, however, bleeding problems are so severe the IUD must be removed. Between 5 and 15 percent of women have their IUD removed during the first year because of excessive bleeding or spotting.

Heavier-than-normal periods may cause iron deficiency anemia and the need for iron supplements. If you normally have painful or heavy periods, you may want to choose the Progestasert or avoid the IUD altogether. The Progestasert can lighten periods and reduce cramps because of the effect of its progesterone on the lining of the uterus.

Cramping and Pain. The most common reaction of the uterus to the presence of the IUD is cramps, very much like strong menstrual cramps, as the uterus tries to expel the device. The cramps can last for a day or two after the insertion and may recur during the first few menstrual periods. Acetaminophen, ibuprofen, and other over-the-counter or prescription painkillers generally can ease this discomfort.

GETTING AN IUD

Have all your questions answered before you have an IUD inserted and be sure it is put in by an experienced professional.

Choosing a Practitioner

Since careful IUD insertion is the key to safety, you want a health care provider who has been properly trained and has had a lot of experience inserting IUDs. Check carefully to find someone who has such qualifications, because IUDs were not widely used in the U.S. from the late 1970s to the late 1980s, when ParaGard came on the market. Many health care providers may not be familiar with IUD insertion and may not feel comfortable suggesting it. IUDs are inserted by physicians, nurse practitioners, physician assistants, and other health care providers working in private medical offices or family planning centers, state and community health department clinics, or in the gynecology department of your hospital. It may be necessary to call a number of such places to find someone experienced in inserting an IUD and providing counseling about it. If sources in your community do not offer this contraceptive, they may be able to refer you to a clinic or health care provider in another community who does.

Before you receive an IUD, you will be asked to read and initial a detailed patient information booklet that outlines the pros and cons of the type of IUD you have chosen. To reduce possible complications, especially from STDs, detailed counseling on IUDs has become an important part of this method. Health care professionals now realize that the success of any method is enhanced when the method is appropriate and counseling has been given about its benefits and possible side effects.

A practitioner will take an extensive medical and sexual history from you. You should not ask for this method if you are likely to have more than one sexual partner, if your partner may have other lovers, or if you have had PID. You will also be given a physical exam, including a Pap smear. Tests for pregnancy and for STDs, particularly chlamydia and gonorrhea, may be a routine part of this exam. After the results are available, you will be given an appointment for the insertion.

When to Have an IUD Inserted

You can have an IUD inserted almost any time, as long as you have not had unprotected intercourse since your last period. Your practitioner may prefer to insert it during your menstrual period, to be certain you are not pregnant. Furthermore, the IUD is easier to insert then, because your cervix is dilated and lubricated by blood, and you are less likely to be bothered by the spotting that insertion usually causes. On the other hand, there is a slightly greater risk of infection and a slightly greater chance of the IUD being expelled when the procedure is done during menstruation. Inserting the IUD at midcycle—at the time of ovulation—can be just as easy as during your period because the cervix is dilated also at that time.

Most practitioners recommend insertion no sooner than six weeks after the delivery of a baby, to avoid the risk of the IUD being expelled as the uterus slowly returns to normal size. It is also possible to have an IUD inserted immediately after childbirth, right after the placenta has passed, although this seldom is done in the United States. An IUD will not interfere with the production or quality of breast milk. The device also can be inserted immediately or within three weeks after an uncomplicated, first trimester abortion, whether spontaneous or induced.

The Insertion Procedure

Before the IUD is inserted you may be given acetaminophen or ibuprofen, to help ease the cramps that can occur when the IUD is inserted.

During insertion, the vagina is held open with a speculum, the same instrument used for examinations of the cervix. The cervix and vagina are cleansed with antiseptic solution. The cervix is held steady with a grasping instrument, the tenaculum, which may cause discomfort or pain when it is first applied. If you are worried about this, ask your provider to apply a bit of local anesthetic to the cervix. The practitioner then guides a skinny, flexible, measuring rod, called the "sound," through the cervical opening to the top of the uterus, to measure its depth and determine which way and how much the uterus may be slanted. The uterus may cramp while the sound is inserted and withdrawn.

The IUD is prepacked into a slim, plastic tube ready for use. The tube slides into the uterus as close to the top as possible. Then the tube is slowly withdrawn, allowing the arms of the T to unfold within the broadest part of the uterus. The inserter is slipped out of the uterus, leaving the IUD in the uterus and the threads in the vagina, where they are clipped to the right length—long enough so you can feel them but not so long they get in the way of a tampon. They are so fine they're impossible to feel during sex. It is a good idea for you to check the location of the threads before you leave the examining room so you know where they are and what they feel like.

Before you leave, you may want to make an appointment for a followup visit a month or so later, so your provider can check to see if your IUD has stayed in the right position.

The reaction of women to the insertion process varies, ranging from none to slight discomfort to a great deal of pain. Most women find the process no more painful than strong menstrual cramps. If you are particularly sensitive to pain, the cervix can be desensitized with a lidocaine injection. Some bleeding may occur after the insertion.

After Your IUD Has Been Inserted

You will not feel the IUD. Neither you nor your partner will be aware of the IUD, because it is in your uterus and not in your vagina. This is a major benefit of this method. You can have intercourse as soon after the insertion as you wish. If you do become aware of the IUD, it may have been partially expelled from the uterus and you need to call your health care provider right away—and use another contraceptive. If your partner can feel the threads, they can be shortened by your practitioner.

Check the strings. The first few months after you have received your IUD is the peak time for it to be expelled. While you are still on the examining table, ask your practitioner to teach you how to check for the threads. If you are familiar with their length, you will notice if that length changes. During the first weeks, check the threads once or twice a week, especially right after your period. If at any time they seem longer or you cannot feel them at all, or if you can feel the IUD itself in your cervix or vagina, call your practitioner immediately. And, if you have sex, use your backup birth control. Aerobics, jogging, or other vigorous physical activities will not dislodge an IUD. The contractions of your uterus during menstruation are the likeliest cause of your IUD being expelled, and the chance of this happening will decrease as time passes.

Be aware of the possibility of infection. Do not forget that if you develop the symptoms of infection mentioned earlier, you should contact your health care provider immediately.

Watch for your menstrual periods. If the IUD has been expelled or has perforated your uterus, it will not provide protection against pregnancy. If your menstrual period does not arrive at all, or if it is late and then is very light, contact your practitioner to check on the possibility of pregnancy.

Heavier periods are common. With the ParaGard, you are likely to have more bleeding, cramps that are more severe, an increase in mucus discharge, and spotting between periods. These disturbances are not unusual with an IUD and they begin to subside after a few months as your uterus gets used to the IUD. If you are anemic, however, those heavier periods could exacerbate the anemia. Discuss this with your health care provider before deciding on this method. If you choose the ParaGard and your periods remain heavy for more than several months, you may wish to switch to a Progestasert.

If you change partners. If you change sex partners or your partner stops being monogamous, start using a barrier method of contraception such as the female condom, diaphragm, cervical cap, or male condom. If your new relationship becomes lasting and mutually monogamous, and you both test free of STDs and HIV infection, you may be able to give up condoms and rely on your IUD for pregnancy protection. Discuss this change with your health care provider, and remember that an STD or HIV may not produce any symptoms.

Tampons and douching. You can wear a tampon without concern while you have an IUD. The IUD is in your uterus, out of reach of any tampon or anything else you put in your vagina. Although douching liquids usually stay in the vagina, douching is not a recommended practice today. It may wash bacteria or sperm up into the uterus.

Additional contraception. The IUD is effective as soon as it is in place. As with any birth control method, however, it is always wise to keep another type of contraceptive on hand in case of emergencies. If the IUD string changes in length or you have another reason to suspect that it is no longer in the right place, start using your backup method right away and call your health care provider.

Have your IUD checked by your health care provider at least once a year.

If you miss a period or have other signs of pregnancy such as tender breasts, call your practitioner right away. If you are pregnant, your IUD should be removed immediately.

You will notice how frequently we stress that you contact your health care provider as soon as you have any negative reaction to your IUD. There is a reason for this. A review of the problems associated with IUDs during the 1970s reveals that early treatment would have prevented many serious complications. Many women who experienced discomfort believed it was typical of the IUD and did not tell their physicians. As a result, many infections and other complications were not treated and the consequences for some were serious.

Removing the IUD

The removal process is much simpler than the insertion. The best time to have an IUD removed is during a menstrual period or during the midcycle days, when the cervix is dilated. In an uncomplicated removal, the practitioner pulls steadily on the threads and slowly draws the IUD from the uterus.

In the uncommon instances when this technique does not work, the cervix may need to be dilated to ease the removal. An anesthetic can be injected into the cervix to reduce pain. If you have worn your IUD for several years, it may be embedded securely in the uterus, or your cervical canal may have narrowed, making the device more difficult and more painful to remove. If the string has worked its way up into the cervix, a long, narrow forceps can be used to get it. A forceps or other slender instrument (IUD hook) can be used to find and withdraw either the threads or the IUD.

NOTE: *Do not* try to remove the IUD yourself or even attempt to tug on the string—if you pull at the wrong angle, you can cut or otherwise injure your cervix.

COST

The average cost of having an IUD inserted ranges from $300 to $700 or more, a cost that should include the device itself, counseling, a physical exam, the necessary tests, and the insertion. Followup visits may be extra. The cost of IUD removal is usually the same as a routine office visit—between $40 and $100. Some Planned Parenthood and other nonprofit family planning clinics make contraceptives like the IUD available on a sliding scale based on their client's income. Some clinics accept Medicaid payments for both insertion and removal.

Since prices for contraceptive services can vary widely even in the same city or state, it is worthwhile to shop around by telephone to find both a good price and an experienced practitioner.

Although the cost of an IUD insertion may seem high, with the ParaGard this one-time expense provides 10 years of contraception. For example, over 10 years a $500 IUD insertion averages out to a yearly cost of $50, much less than the typical annual expense of the Pill, condoms, or spermicide products. Consequently, the copper IUD is one of the least expensive methods of birth control for those who use it for many years.

PART FOUR

Surgical Methods

12

Female Sterilization: Tubal Occlusion

Healthy women may remain fertile until their late 40s, and healthy men are fertile all their lives. Most couples have all the children they want long before they lose their fertility. As a result, they face a good many years in which they have to use some effective form of birth control. Many couples choose sterilization as a solution. As a result, voluntary sterilization is one of the most common contraceptive methods used in the United States. Either partner can be sterilized to end the possibility of conception.

Female sterilization involves permanently closing off (occluding) the fallopian tubes to prevent sperm from reaching an egg. This is done surgically.

One of the most effective contraceptive methods available, female sterilization has a failure rate of less than 2 percent in preventing pregnancy over a 10-year period. The risk of pregnancy is even smaller for women age 28 and older. The greatest failure risk occurs among women under age 28, who tend to be more sexually active and more fertile.

If you have your tubes "tied," you will continue to produce female hormones and to menstruate as usual, and your sexual functioning is unaffected. The surgery will not change your skin, breasts, or weight, nor does it affect the vagina, uterus, or ovaries. An egg cell is still released by the ovaries every month and enters the nearby fallopian tube. The egg cell stops, however, where the tube has been closed off, disintegrates, and is absorbed by the body.

Sterilization surgery can be performed with a local anesthetic or under general anesthesia. At some medical centers the most commonly used methods—laparoscopy and minilaparotomy—are performed on an outpatient basis, using a local anesthetic and mild sedatives. Both these procedures usually take less than 30 minutes. When local anesthesia is used, most women are able to go home after an hour or two of resting in the recovery room. If a general or spinal anesthetic is used, it may be necessary to stay in the clinic or hospital a bit longer.

The type of surgery used depends on when the procedure is done, on your health and medical condition, and on the policies and preferences of the surgeon, the medical center, and the patient. If the sterilization is performed immediately after childbirth, a minilaparotomy is preferred because this approach is easiest when the uterus and tubes are high in the abdomen, as they are right after a childbirth. It is called a *minilaparotomy* because the incision is less than 2 inches long. When tubes are tied at another time, the surgical technique used is most often a laparoscopy.

If you are overweight, have adhesions from previous abdominal surgery, or have an abdominal abnormality, you are likely to need a somewhat more complicated procedure. You should choose a skilled gynecologist/surgeon and a fully equipped medical center. Although it may be possible to carry out the operation with local anesthesia, general anesthesia should be available in case it is needed. Just which technique will be used depends on the preferences and experience of the patient and surgeon.

METHODS AND TECHNIQUES

Two methods are used to reach the fallopian tubes in order to close them.

IN A NUTSHELL

FEMALE STERILIZATION

Sterilization is a permanent form of birth control. For women, being sterilized means that the two tubes that carry eggs from the ovary to the uterus are tied shut, or cut, or blocked in some other way. This prevents sperm from reaching the egg to fertilize it. It is extremely effective.

Having your tubes tied does not affect your hormones. It does not change your menstrual cycle or your feelings about sex. Only the tubes are changed. Your vagina, uterus, and ovaries remain the same. Your breasts, skin, and weight are not affected.

Sterilization surgery usually takes about 30 minutes. If a local anesthetic is used, you can go home after an hour or two of rest at the clinic. If a general anesthetic or spinal is used, the recovery time may be somewhat longer.

The surgery is done through very small incisions in the belly that require only one or two stitches. It can be done in the hospital right after having a baby, or at any time.

Because it is permanent, this method of birth control is not advised for young women whose lives may change so they want to have another child. It is important to think about this very carefully and not to make a decision without getting counseling. Good clinics, hospitals, and doctors who perform sterilizations always offer counseling.

Sterilization does not protect against STDs of any kind.

Minilaparotomy

In a minilaparotomy, an approximately 2-inch incision is made low in the abdomen, often just above the pubic hair, where it will not be very obvious. Using an instrument placed in the uterus via the vagina, the surgeon gently pushes the uterus and fallopian tubes up to the abdominal wall to make it easier to reach the tubes through the incision. The surgeon then uses a special hook, a forceps, or a finger to reach in and lift out a loop of fallopian tube.

The tube is closed off by the application of a high-frequency electric current (electrocoagulation), a plastic ring, or a special spring clip. Some surgeons use a suture to tie the tube in a loop, and then remove the loop itself. After both tubes have been closed off or tied and replaced in the abdomen, the incision is shut with a few stitches.

The minilap is the method favored when women have a tubal occlusion right after childbirth. As we mentioned, this is a good time to perform an occlusion, from a surgical point of view. The uterus and tubes are high in the abdomen and easier to reach. A minilap cannot be done if a women is very overweight, however. The extra layers of fatty abdominal tissue require a larger incision, and the procedure becomes a regular laparotomy (abdominal surgery).

Laparoscopy

Laparoscopy is the method most frequently used today in the U.S. and Europe for female sterilization. When performed by a surgeon experienced in the technique, it is extremely safe. Today it is often done as an outpatient procedure, which can reduce its cost.

Instead of requiring a conventional incision, laparoscopy is performed through one or two punctures into the abdomen. A hollow needle is inserted into the site to inflate the abdomen with gas, usually nitrous oxide or carbon dioxide, which expands the abdominal cavity and lifts the wall of the belly away from the structures within it. The needle is then withdrawn and a sharp-pointed trocar is used to make a puncture into the abdomen for the long, slender

ISSUES TO CONSIDER BEFORE STERILIZATION

- Vasectomy (male sterilization) is simpler, safer, and less expensive than female sterilization. If both vasectomy and sterilization are equally acceptable to a couple, vasectomy is the medically preferred procedure.
- It is not a legal requirement to have the permission of a spouse in order to undergo sterilization.
- Persons who wish to be sterilized must be legally competent to make this decision, which usually means being over age 21 and mentally competent. If federal funds are paying for sterilization, after signing a consent form for voluntary surgical contraception, women (and men having vasectomies) must wait 30 days before having the surgery. These include sterilizations paid for by the U.S. Department of Health and Human Services (Medicaid) or performed in U.S. Public Health, military, or Indian Health Service facilities.

laparoscope. The laparoscope wand contains a light source for illuminating the inside of the abdomen and a lens through which the surgeon can view it. There are many variations of this technique, and your surgeon may use a procedure that is slightly different.

If the operation is a single-puncture laparoscopy, the operating instruments enter the abdomen through the operating channel of the laparoscope (Figure 12.1). They are used both to grasp and close each fallopian tube in turn, guided by the surgeon's view through the scope. In a double-puncture approach, the operating instruments are inserted in the second incision, while the surgeon uses the scope at the original incision to guide their movements.

After the tubes have been closed with silicone rubber bands, electrocoagulation, spring clips, or a suture tie, the organs in the abdomen are inspected through the scope to make sure there has been no injury or bleeding caused by the procedure. The laparoscope then is removed, the gas expelled from the abdomen, and the incision closed with a suture or two. The only protective covering needed for each tiny incision is a small bandage. If any gas remains, it may cause some abdominal or shoulder discomfort, but it dissipates in a few days.

Occlusion Methods

Probably the most common technique for closing off the fallopian tubes during laparoscopic sterilization is electrocoagulation. A high-frequency electric current is applied very briefly to the narrow, middle section of the tube. The current heats the tissue, causing scars to develop at the site, permanently blocking the tube. It also kills the nerves at the site, so there is less discomfort after the surgery. Safest, most effective, and most commonly used is bipolar electrocoagulation. The bipolar instrument looks like a tiny set of tongs. The current passes down one tong, through the tissue of the tube, and up the other tong, effectively limiting the burned tissue to the small area held between the tongs.

The method most frequently used during a minilap is ligation, using a suture to tie each tube and then removing the section of the tube between the ties. Many surgeons prefer the Pomeroy technique,

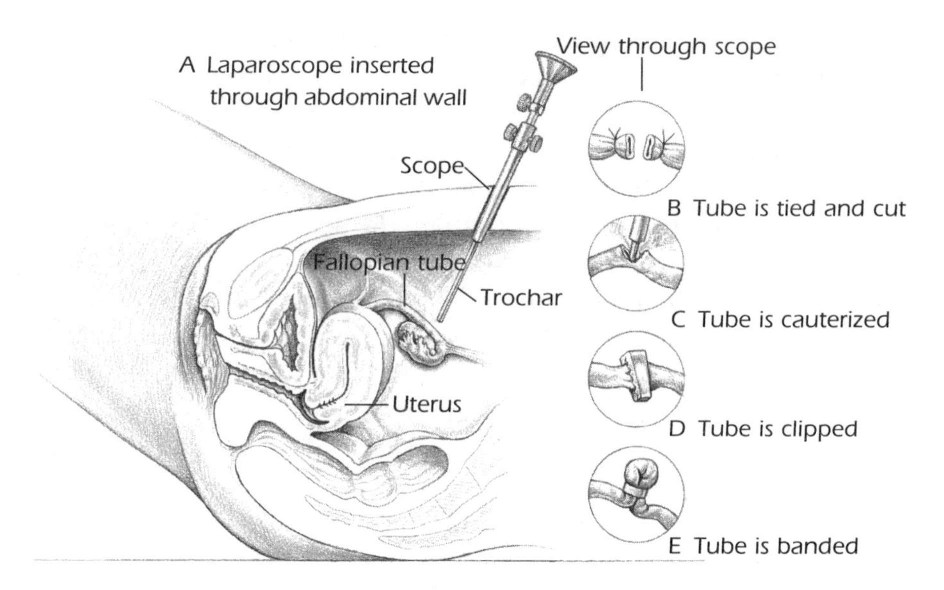

FIGURE 12.1 Laparoscopy and Various Tubal Ligation Methods

in which the tube is tied tightly in a loop and then the loop portion is snipped off.

The oviducts also can be blocked by pinching them shut with mechanical devices, such as metal or plastic clips or small, silastic rings that are like strong, long-lasting rubber bands. These devices fasten tightly around the fallopian tube, holding it in an immovable grasp. Eventually the pinched tissue dies, forming a permanent seal. These clips and rings have the advantage of damaging only the tissue in their immediate vicinity. They are likely to cause several hours of postoperative cramping, however, because of the pressure put on the tube.

Although most tubal occlusions have been performed as hospital inpatient procedures, there now is an increasing trend for these to be outpatient procedures. *When done in an outpatient setting, it is important that the clinic or other facility have formal ties with a nearby hospital, in case an emergency occurs during the procedure.* Certain conditions discovered during the surgery—such as adhesions from undiagnosed endometriosis—can make it necessary to stop the operation and repeat it later at a full-facility hospital. Insurance plans frequently cover the cost of sterilization.

Local Versus General Anesthesia

Local anesthesia for laparoscopic sterilization is effective in preventing pain. Local anesthesia is particularly appropriate for a minilaparotomy or a laparoscopy, because these procedures cause little trauma to the tissues and take a short time to execute. Short-term, general anesthesia, which means the patient sleeps, also is used.

Local anesthesia involves injecting a drug into the area being treated to interrupt the function of the pain-carrying nerves, making the area insensitive to pain. You are awake but usually given a sedative for relaxation and relief of anxiety. The use of local anesthesia has several advantages: (1) it avoids risking the complications that can occur with general anesthesia; (2) for most patients it means a shorter recovery time and less time at the clinic or hospital; and (3) it may reduce the cost of the operation.

Using a local anesthetic means the gynecologist must make changes in how he or she executes the surgery. Having you awake but sedated makes it necessary to perform the surgery more gently. Furthermore, the physician must be in continual communication with you, telling you what is being done and what sensations or discomfort to expect as the fallopian tubes and other organs are manipulated. Occasionally, you will have to be warned not to move. A local anesthetic eliminates the pain, but you may still experience some discomfort.

General anesthesia, by contrast, induces a loss of consciousness and sensation, usually by injected or inhaled drugs. You feel nothing, which helps the surgeon carry out the procedure with dispatch. Nevertheless, general anesthesia is associated with many possible complications: low blood pressure, irregular heartbeat, heart attack, airway obstruction, allergic reactions, brain damage, and death. Although these reactions are rare, general anesthesia should be used only when necessary.

Epidural and spinal blocks are forms of regional anesthesia. With these techniques, the nerves are anesthetized where they branch from the spinal cord. These can be used for childbirth and abdominal surgery, and some gynecologists now use them for sterilization.

Each type of anesthesia has its advantages and disadvantages. Discuss them all with your gynecologist/surgeon. If you prefer a local, you may have to make some inquiries to find a clinic or hospital that favors this method or offers a choice, although it is more widely used today because it is less expensive. In some communities, however, you may find that the only available gynecologist prefers using general anesthesia.

EFFECTIVENESS AND REVERSIBILITY

Sterilization is extremely effective and should be considered permanent. It is possible to repair occluded fallopian tubes so that they can function again, but this is major surgery and does not always work.

Failure Rate

As we noted, female sterilization is more than 98 percent effective over a 10-year period. Failures happen because an occluding device did not work properly, for example, a spring clip that does not exert sufficient pressure, or because electrocoagulation was not complete. A channel also can re-form in an incompletely sealed tube, allowing eggs or sperm to pass through and meet. Failure also can occur if the surgery is not performed carefully or a structure other than the tube was occluded.

Reversibility

Never contemplate having a tubal occlusion with the idea that someday you might want to have it reversed. Life situations can change unexpectedly and unpredictable events can lead to the desire for a child. Divorce and remarriage, a change in career plans, an alteration in your emotional or financial status, or the death of a child can create a strong wish to reverse an occlusion. Women under the age of 30, particularly, are advised against a tubal occlusion, because younger women are more likely to experience life changes.

If there is even the slightest chance that you might want a child in the future, use a reversible type of contraception.

Because of the possibility of regret after an irreversible procedure, careful counseling is important before sterilization. Counseling is available from physicians and family planning clinics, and no tubal occlusion should be performed without it.

Tubal occlusions can be reversed only under the best of circumstances. Reversal does not always lead to pregnancy, because delicate microsurgery is necessary to reverse the blockage of the tubes.

Sterilization procedures that destroy too much of the tube or remove the fimbria, the part of the tube that collects the released egg cell, make a reversal impossible. And it is not unusual for a surgeon to start a reversal procedure only to find that, in addition to the deliberate scarring caused by the occlusion method, the woman's tubes have been harmed by the adhesions and scarring of undiagnosed pelvic inflammatory disease or endometriosis.

For a reversal to be successful, you need to have healthy fallopian tubes that were damaged minimally during sterilization. To become pregnant, you also need to be ovulating and have a fertile partner.

Chances for reversing a sterilization are best if a clip or silastic band was used to occlude the tubes. The most effective method, electrocautery, causes more extensive destruction, making it the most difficult to reverse. Some clinicians prefer to occlude the narrowest part of the tube whenever possible, in order to preserve the greatest amount of tissue—just in case the patient someday wants to have her sterilization reversed.

Although microsurgery techniques have increased the possiblity of reversing a tubal occlusion, success rates for this surgery are modest, and the expense is high. Because of age, irregular ovulation, and other fertility problems, a high percentage of sterilized women are not good candidates for a reversal attempt. Before having such an operation, you and your partner should be tested for other fertility problems, and you should have an examination by laparoscopy to determine the condition of your tubes and whether a reversal of the occlusion is feasible.

POSSIBLE COMPLICATIONS

Major complications as a result of female sterilization are infrequent. In the United States, the fatality rate is 4 per 100,000 procedures, mostly from complications from the use of general anesthesia.

Surgical Complications

Complications from the surgery itself can include infection and internal bleeding as the result of an instrument piercing a major blood vessel. Laparoscopic instruments can puncture organs or the intestines and can perforate the uterus. In rare instances, inflating the abdomen leads to a gas bubble in the blood system, which can be immediately fatal. Electrocoagulation instruments, if not managed carefully, can burn tissues other than the fallopian tubes.

Major complications—including injuries that require further surgery to repair—occur in just under 2 out of every 1,000 patients. The overall rate for major and minor complications is approximately 6 percent of the laparoscopies performed.

After having a tubal occlusion, be alert for such symptoms as fever, severe or persistent pain in the abdomen, or bleeding from the incision. These could indicate an infection or an injury that occurred as a result of the surgery. Complications can be minimized if they are treated right away, so bring such symptoms immediately to the attention of the gynecologist who performed the operation. Injuries made by the instruments usually require laparotomy to repair.

The risk of complications from laparoscopy is influenced considerably by the skills of the surgeon. The clinician who performs any sterilization surgery, particularly laparoscopy, should have special training in it. Furthermore, experience plays an important part—gynecologists who do fewer than 100 laparoscopies each year have a much higher rate of complications.

Ectopic Pregnancy

Although tubal occlusions rarely fail, if you become pregnant after being sterilized, there is a considerable chance the embryo will lodge itself in the fallopian tube. Anytime you feel any signs of pregnancy after sterilization, such as morning sickness, tender breasts, or no menstrual period, contact your physician for a pregnancy test.

If the pregnancy is ectopic, you may develop these symptoms:

- Sudden, severe, or persistent abdominal pain or cramping, often on one side.
- Unusual vaginal bleeding or spotting, along with abdominal pain, especially if this occurs after an unusually light period, or a late or missed period.
- A spell of faintness or dizziness (an indication of internal bleeding) together with any of the preceding symptoms.

If you have these symptoms and *cannot* reach your doctor, seek help at the nearest hospital emergency room. A pregnancy in a fallopian tube may rupture at any time, creating an emergency situation.

Although ectopic pregnancy is a potential complication of sterilization, 100,000 women who have had a tubal occlusion will experience fewer ectopic pregnancies than an equal number of unsterilized women who use no contraception.

WHEN TO HAVE A TUBAL OCCLUSION

From a surgical point of view, the easiest time for a woman to be sterilized is immediately after childbirth, when the uterus and fallopian tubes are still high in the abdomen and easier to reach than when they are in their usual lower position. In the past, when sterilizations required hospitalization, this seemed a logical time for the procedure—the woman was already in the hospital; the surgery did not extend the hospital stay; the operation was easier; and so the cost was less.

Today, however, most sterilizations do not need to be performed in a hospital, and many women feel that immediately after childbirth is *not* a good time to have any additional discomfort and pain.

Psychologically, too, while you are pregnant or soon after you have had a baby may be poor times to decide on sterilization. You may be under particular emotional and physical stress at these times and preoccupied with other important issues—especially those relating to the new baby. The decision to have a tubal occlusion should be made when you are able to think clearly about your life. Although you do not need the consent of your spouse in order to be sterilized, it is a good idea to include your partner in the decision-making process.

A tubal occlusion also can be performed immediately after an induced or spontaneous abortion. Because your tubes and uterus are not as enlarged as they are after a full-term pregnancy, either a minilap or a laparoscopy can be used.

Caution must also be exercised regarding sterilization immediately after abortion. Abortion can be an emotional, stressful event. It is not the best time for deciding on a method of contraception that is permanent. Do not choose to be sterilized if you are feeling under any sort of pressure—from yourself or others—to do so.

HAVING A TUBAL OCCLUSION

You can change your mind anytime before the surgery. If you are the least bit uncomfortable with your decision to be sterilized or you are not totally certain about the prospect of having no more children, cancel or postpone the procedure.

Choosing a Practitioner

The most obvious person with whom to discuss the possibility of a tubal occlusion—after your partner—is your obstetrician/gynecologist. Nevertheless, do not assume automatically that he or she should perform the surgery. The more frequently a clinician performs a particular procedure, the safer it will be, so you want to seek out a physician who performs many sterilizations. It is perfectly all right to ask where he or she was trained in laparoscopy and how often he or she now does sterilizations.

If there are not many medical resources where you live, or you are not satisfied with them, call your nearest Planned Parenthood clinic or the gynecology department of the closest medical school or

ARE YOU A GOOD CANDIDATE FOR STERILIZATION?

A tubal occlusion may be right for you if you are sure you do not want to be pregnant at any time in the future—for example, if you have health problems that can make pregnancy unsafe, if you do not want to pass on a hereditary disease or disability, or if you have all the children you want. Sterilization may also be the answer if you and your partner cannot use or do not want to use the reversible contraceptive methods currently available.

teaching hospital and ask for the names of several doctors who are experienced in sterilization. Many hospitals offer this operation, often on an outpatient basis. Some hospitals can offer sterilization because they receive public funds to provide family planning care to low-income families. If you choose a clinic outside a hospital, make certain it has an arrangement with a nearby hospital to provide emergency backup.

This chapter provides only a general outline—each gynecologic surgeon has her or his own approach to tubal occlusion. When you have chosen a surgeon, before your first appointment write down your questions and ask for a step-by-step description of the procedure. Do not be afraid to ask questions, particularly about the possible risks of this surgery. If you want more information after your first visit, ask for it. Sterilization is an important step and should not be undertaken until your questions have been answered to your satisfaction. Make sure you receive the counseling that is a vital part of the process.

Today, before most operations take place, you are asked to sign an informed consent document. In general, the document for a sterilization covers these points: (1) the exact type of operation being performed, including its risks and benefits; (2) the availability of alternative, reversible methods of birth control; (3) the fact that a successful sterilization will prevent you from ever having more children; (4) the failure rate that is possible with this procedure; and (5) the fact that you can change your mind about having the surgery without losing your insurance or medical or financial benefits. The last point is important when the tubal occlusion would be paid for by public funds.

Before and After the Operation

If you are using birth control pills, mention this to your surgeon in case you need to discontinue them before surgery. In this case, be sure to use another contraceptive method until the surgery is complete. If you are pregnant at the time you are scheduled for sterilization, the pregnancy most probably will continue unless you choose to have an abortion as well as the sterilization. An abortion can be performed at the same time.

Do not eat or drink anything 8 hours before the operation. Take a bath or shower just before you go to the hospital or clinic, and thoroughly wash your abdomen, navel, and pubic area.

Arrange to have someone accompany you home afterward. Because your reflexes will be slowed down, it is not safe for you to drive for some hours after having general anesthesia or the sedatives used with local anesthesia. Plan to have someone with you for the first 24 hours after the surgery.

Plan to rest for at least 24 hours after the procedure and avoid any heavy work or lifting for at least 7 days, to give your body time to heal. Build as much flexibility and rest into your schedule as possible—some women recover more slowly than others from the effects of surgery and anesthesia. It may be a good idea to schedule sterilization surgery for a Thursday or Friday, to gain the weekend days for extra rest.

If you have a minilap or laparoscopy with local anesthesia, you may feel ready to go home as early as an hour after the procedure. If you have general anesthesia, you need to stay a little longer. After such a brief operation, most women recover from general anesthesia after 4 or 5 hours; rarely is an overnight stay in the hospital necessary. If the operation is performed immediately after childbirth, your hospital stay may be lengthened by a day.

If you have general anesthesia, you are likely to feel nauseated, weak, and tired until the next day. Your throat will be sore from the endotracheal tube put into your windpipe.

POSTOPERATIVE DANGER SIGNALS

Although some pain at the site of the incision and some abdominal discomfort are to be expected, any sign of an infection at the incision, any abdominal pain that is not relieved by mild pain medication, or any pain that lasts longer than 12 hours should be brought to the attention of the physician who performed the surgery.

Other symptoms of possible complications include the following:

- Chest pain, shortness of breath, coughing, or feeling faint.
- Fever with a temperature over 100.4 degrees Fahrenheit.
- Blood or fluid coming from the incision after the first day or two.
- Moderate or heavy vaginal bleeding.

After a laparoscopy, you may experience pain in a shoulder—this is caused by the gas used to inflate your abdomen. Although much of the gas is removed after the surgery, enough can remain to cause discomfort for a few days. These effects fade as the gas is absorbed by your body over the next couple of days.

Although the area of the incision is likely to be painful, the discomfort almost always can be relieved by taking a non-aspirin type of pain medication such as acetaminophen. Take one or two tablets every 4 to 6 hours as long as you need pain relief. You may have an occasional feeling of discomfort or aching in your lower abdomen as a result of the manipulation of the uterus or tubes. This usually disappears after a few days.

Some women experience menstrual problems after a tubal occlusion. This effect has been studied by several groups of researchers—with conflicting results. It does appear that some women experience shorter menstrual cycles, greater blood loss, and irregular bleeding after their tubes have been tied. These changes did not happen immediately—most were not noticeable until almost 2 years had passed. Women in the study who had abnormal cycles before sterilization were most likely to have menstrual changes after the procedure.

Tubal occlusion does not protect you against sexually transmitted diseases, including AIDS. Although you are safe from pregnancy, if you are not in a mutually monogamous relationship, you or your partner still need to use a barrier method of contraception, preferably a condom, for STD protection.

COST

The cost of a tubal occlusion varies, depending on the setting in which it is done and on the physician who performs it. The cost ranges from $1,200 to about $3,000. (A high cost does not necessarily guarantee a better quality procedure.) Medicaid, most insurance plans, and most health maintenance organizations pay for sterilization.

• 13 •

Male Sterilization: *Vasectomy*

Vasectomy, the sterilization procedure for men, is simpler and safer than female sterilization and is usually performed in a doctor's office or a clinic. A vasectomy takes approximately 20 minutes, is almost 100 percent effective, has few complications, and is permanent. Some 500,000 vasectomies are performed each year.

The term "vasectomy" means cutting the two vasa deferentia, the sperm ducts, that carry sperm from the testicles to the penis. A small portion of each duct is usually removed and the cut ends are closed off. This procedure effectively prevents sperm from getting into the semen that is ejaculated during sex. Although it is possible to reverse a vasectomy, a reversal procedure requires difficult microsurgery. Under the best conditions, the reversal succeeds only about 50 percent of the time (a pregnancy is viewed as success), and it is very expensive.

A vasectomy does not influence a man's virility, nor does it have any negative impact on his overall health. It does not lead to premature aging, and the most recent studies find that it does not increase the chance of prostate cancer. After a vasectomy, a man still produces male hormones, has erections and orgasms, and ejaculates. Even the amount of fluid that he ejaculates is virtually unchanged, since sperm contribute only a small amount—3 to 5 percent—to the total volume.

The only change that takes place is that the semen contains no sperm, so it cannot cause a pregnancy. In fact, some men report an increase in sexual desire after having a vasectomy, because they are no longer worried about the possibility of an unwanted pregnancy.

After your vasectomy you will still be fertile for a while, until all the sperm that were present when the surgery was performed have been ejaculated or have died. This process takes between 2 and 4 months—or about 20 ejaculations. Meanwhile, you or your partner should use another contraceptive method until two consecutive specimens of semen are found to be free of sperm.

A vasectomy does not protect either partner against AIDS or other sexually transmitted diseases.

METHODS

The standard vasectomy technique uses a tiny incision; the "no-scalpel" method utilizes a puncture.

Standard Vasectomy

The vasa deferentia that carry sperm from the testicles to the pe-

IN A NUTSHELL

VASECTOMY

Vasectomy is a permanent form of birth control for men. The tubes that carry the sperm from the testicles to the penis are cut and the cut ends are closed off. This prevents sperm from getting into the semen that is ejaculated during sex.

This method of birth control is highly effective and has few complications. It is faster, simpler, and less expensive than female sterilization.

A vasectomy does not change your virility or strength or increase your chance of prostate cancer. You still produce male hormones, have erections, and ejaculate.

A local anesthetic is injected near the sperm tubes in the testicles. A tiny incision is made. Each tube is pulled through the incision, cut, and tied off. The whole operation takes about 20 minutes. The incision is so small it does not need stitches.

Vasectomies are done as outpatient procedures at doctor's offices, clinics, and hospitals.

A vasectomy does not protect either partner against STDs, including AIDS.

nis can be felt just under the skin of the scrotum. The outer, muscular wall of each sperm duct is thick and less flexible than the nearby blood vessels, which are soft and pliable to the touch (Figure 13.1). The physician doing the vasectomy uses his or her fingers or a special clamp to hold one vas firmly under the skin while injecting a local anesthetic, usually lidocaine. (The injection hurts for several seconds.) Some practitioners apply a second injection just above the vasectomy site to act as a nerve block for more complete protection against pain.

When the area is numb, the doctor uses a surgical clamp to hold the skin tightly over the vas, making a tiny (1/4 to 1/2 inch) incision through the skin and the thin layer of muscle tissue. When the duct is accessible, a very small forceps or similar instrument is used to pull it gently up through the incision. Although the site of the surgery itself is anesthetized, you may still feel a pulling sensation on the upper part of the duct.

Many clinicians prefer to make an incision directly over each duct, but some make a single incision halfway between them and

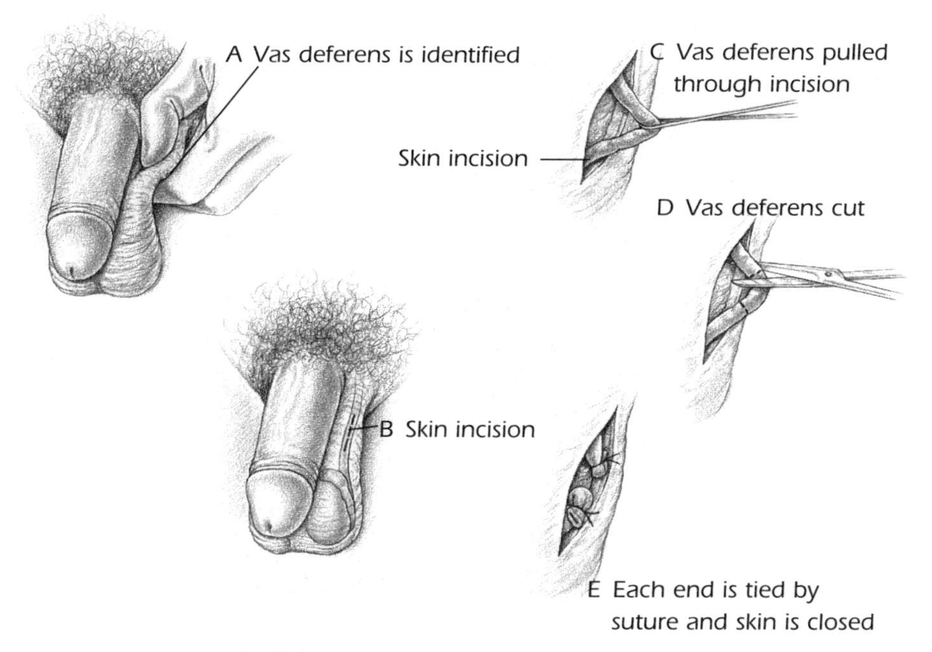

FIGURE 13.1 Standard Vasectomy Procedure

draw each duct over to the opening to snip it. After each vas has been severed and its cut ends closed, it is returned to the scrotum. The incision is closed with an absorbable suture—some incisions are so small they need no suture.

To sever the vas, the surgeon may snip through it with scissors and then remove a short bit of tube to make certain the two cut ends will not join again accidently. Because the human body has such a strong tendency to repair itself, most physicians today seal the cut ends with electrocautery, employing a technique similar to the one used in female sterilization to close the fallopian tubes. A quick touch of high-frequency electric current causes the inside of the duct to scar into a permanent seal. Other methods include folding and suturing each severed end back on itself, or suturing a bit of the outside sheath of the duct over the end to close it.

Sperm will still be produced by the testicle and may build up behind the closed end of the duct that carries them from the testicle. Accumulated sperm sometimes—rarely—can be painful. Fortunately, they have a short life cycle and soon die off and are absorbed by the body.

Some surgeons may leave open the end of the duct that carries sperm from the testicle—the epididymis—closing only the section that connects with the penis. This allows sperm to spill and not accumulate in the delicate epididymis. A vasectomy that leaves the epididymis portion of the vas open avoids the possibility of the epididymis being harmed by pressure from accumulated sperm. Regardless of where sperm go, however, they are absorbed. Although a vasectomy that closes off only one end of the dissected vas may be more reversible, it also has a somewhat greater chance of failing.

A vasectomy usually takes about 20 minutes. After a brief recovery period at the clinic, it is advisable to rest in bed at home for 24 hours to allow the incisions to heal. You may experience a dull, aching pain and some bleeding for a few days. You can take a painkiller, preferably one that does not contain aspirin, such as acetaminophen, because aspirin reduces the blood's ability to clot. Men who do physical labor generally are advised to wait a week before going back to strenuous work, in order to encourage healing and avoid bleeding complications. All men who have had vasectomies should wear an athletic supporter or jockey shorts for four to six weeks to support the scrotum until it is completely healed.

No-Scalpel Vasectomy

A vasectomy procedure that is growing in popularity is the no-scalpel method, which was developed in China in the 1970s. It is called the "no-scalpel" method because a puncture instead of an incision is made in the scrotum to reach the sperm ducts. A puncture instead of an incision greatly reduces the risk of accidently cutting into a blood vessel. The approach takes only about 10 minutes and causes considerably less soreness, bleeding, and bruising afterward. Furthermore, the chance of infection or a hematoma (a collection of blood) is much less.

As in a standard vasectomy, some clinicians are using the anesthesia technique that is basically a nerve block. A small amount of local anesthetic is injected at the site in the scrotum where the puncture will be made and then, with the same needle, additional anesthetic is injected near the vasal nerve above the vasectomy site. The anesthetic takes effect almost immediately. When the area is numb, a sharp instrument is used to pierce the skin of the scrotum and the vas sheath where the duct is most prominent and accessible beneath the skin. The same instrument is then used to spread apart the opening. Each vas deferens is pulled, in turn, through this tiny opening, cut, and closed off according to usual vasectomy practice (Figure 13.2). After each duct is closed, it is put back in place in the scrotum. No stitches are required to close the wound. The puncture contracts and becomes almost invisible. Antibiotic ointment is applied and the area covered with a small gauze bandage that is held in place with the help of a snug pair of undershorts or an athletic supporter.

EFFECTIVENESS AND REVERSIBILITY

Vasectomy is highly effective and should not be considered a reversible method. Although it is possible to repair the occluded sperm ducts, this requires delicate surgery and does not always succeed.

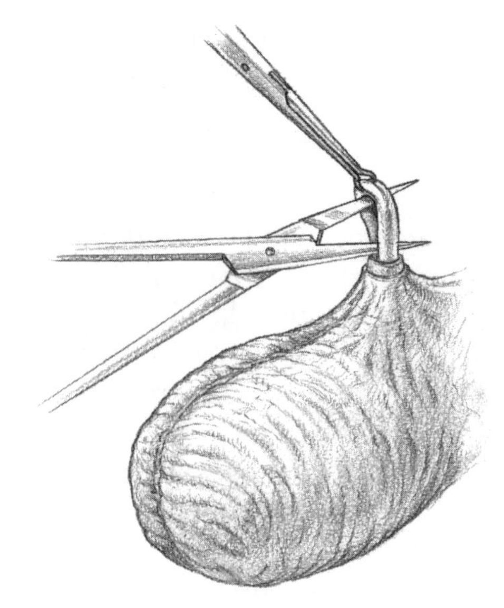

FIGURE 13.2 No-Scalpel Vasectomy

Failure Rate

A typical first-year failure rate for vasectomy is 0.5 to 1.0 percent. A true failure of the technique can take place only when a closed duct opens or reconnects, or when a structure other than the duct—such as a blood vessel—is mistakenly cut and closed off instead of the vas. Such events are very rare.

Pregnancies can occur if you have unprotected intercourse before your reproductive tract has been totally emptied of the sperm that were present when the surgery was performed. In a few extremely rare cases, men who had at least two negative sperm counts after a vasectomy fathered children.

Reversibility

Like tubal occlusions in women, vasectomies sometimes can be reversed successfully. The success of a reversal procedure depends largely on the skill of the surgeon. The diameter of the inner canal of the vas deferens has been described as being approximately the diameter of a pinpoint. To achieve a clear connection between the two severed ends of the duct, the surgeon must use a microscope while rejoining the ends of these almost invisible tubes. Because this operation is major surgery, it calls for the use of general anesthesia, is expensive, and requires a long recovery time.

If the epididymis has been damaged, the injured area of this fine, tightly coiled tube must be bypassed by suturing the end of the vas to the nearest healthy part of the epididymis. Since the epididymis is even more delicate than the inner canal of the vas, this sort of repair often fails. Moreover, it may take months or even years before an epididymis long dilated by sperm buildup finally returns to normal functioning.

Pregnancy rates following a reversal procedure vary widely, from 16 percent to 79 percent, with the majority of clinics achieving a success rate close to 50 percent of couples who passed a screening process for possible success. For all practical purposes, vasectomy should be viewed as a permanent form of contraception.

HEALTH EFFECTS

Complications after vasectomy occur only in a small fraction of the procedures. They include:

Hematoma. The most common complication from a vasectomy is a hematoma, a mass of clotted blood, caused by damage to a blood vessel during the surgery. Normally, blood drains from the incision, but occasionally the blood accumulates instead of draining, and within 24 hours the scrotum becomes enlarged and painful. Draining this may require a brief hospitalization. Although unpleasant, hematomas generally do not cause permanent harm. They may be prevented if you spend the first 24 to 48 hours off your feet, preferably in bed. Any upright activity, even walking, increases pressure on the blood vessels and the likelihood of a hematoma. In a review of almost 25,000 vasectomies, hematomas occurred in 1.6 percent.

Infection. An infection occasionally develops near the site of the incision. It should be treated immediately with antibiotics. Infections occur in 1.5 to 3.4 percent of vasectomies.

ARE YOU A GOOD CANDIDATE FOR VASECTOMY?

Vasectomy is an excellent contraceptive option for the man who is in a stable relationship and has all the children he wants. Men whose partners have health problems that may make a pregnancy unsafe frequently turn to vasectomy as the most reliable form of birth control. Similarly, couples who are at risk for passing on a hereditary disease or disability often choose sterilization—and vasectomy is the safer and less expensive form.

If you are young, are not sure about having children, or are considering sterilization in the hope that not having to worry about birth control might steady your relationship, you are not a likely candidate for vasectomy. If you are thinking of storing your sperm in case you may want children in the future, vasectomy is probably not for you at this time. (Sperm banking is expensive and not always successful.) Finally, if you have any reservations at all about vasectomy or if you are under any pressure to have the procedure, postpone the decision.

Epididymitis. Acute inflammation of the epididymis occasionally follows vasectomy surgery. It is treated with heat, support of the scrotum to relieve discomfort, and antibiotics. Epididymitis occurs in approximately 1.4 percent of vasectomies.

Sperm Granulomas. A painful nodule or lump can develop at the site of the vasectomy or in the epididymis. This is a sperm granuloma (a localized inflammatory reaction), usually caused by the presence of sperm that have leaked from one of the severed ducts. The lumps rarely become painful—only if the lump touches a nerve. This problem occurs in about 0.3 percent of vasectomies and only needs treatment if it is painful. Treatment may require having the vas deferens on that side removed so sperm will no longer reach the granuloma. The lump then is absorbed by the body and stops causing pain.

HAVING A VASECTOMY

Because it is difficult to reverse a vasectomy successfully, choosing it should be given long, careful thought.

Changing Your Mind

Before undergoing this operation, it is essential that you feel comfortable with the fact that a vasectomy is permanent. If you have any doubts, postpone the operation until you are more certain of your feelings, and have gotten all the information you feel you need. Other men who have had vasectomies can provide you with useful insights and advice. Family planning clinics may do much better than individual physicians in providing information and counseling. Do not hesitate to ask a lot of questions.

Choosing a Practitioner

Urologists, family physicians, and general surgeons perform vasectomies. Your own family health care provider or your partner's gynecologist are good places to start making inquiries. In addition, most hospitals have at least one physician on staff—usually a urologist—who is experienced in both the standard and no-scalpel procedures. If medical resources are scarce in your area, get in touch with a local family planning clinic, Visiting Nurse Association, health department, or county medical society. (Family planning clinics often are listed in the Yellow Pages.) Or contact the Association for Voluntary Surgical Contraception, 79 Madison Avenue, New York, N.Y. 10016 (212-561-8000). The association is an especially helpful resource if you are interested in the no-scalpel vasectomy and finding a practitioner who has experience with it.

Vasectomies and Pain

No matter which technique is used, some men find vasectomy painful. Before the surgery, make certain you understand exactly how your physician plans to perform the procedure and what he will do to minimize the possibility of pain and discomfort. Pain tends to be magnified when it is unexpected, so knowing every detail of the operation goes a long way toward making the surgery more comfortable. A sedative beforehand also makes things easier. As mentioned earlier, an additional injection of anesthetic above the site of the incision or puncture may be more effective in blocking pain along the vasal nerve, which carries sensation to the vasa deferentia. This approach is worth discussing with your doctor.

Before the Operation

Your doctor will conduct a physical examination beforehand that will take into account the existence of any local infections, hernias, and the present condition of your testicles and penis. A vasectomy is more difficult if you have an undescended testicle, a hernia or a repaired hernia, or some other abnormality. A health history will note any condition that may affect the surgery and its outcome, such as past operations and illnesses, as well as allergies to local anesthetics and pain medications.

Make arrangements to have someone drive you home afterward, and to avoid all exertion for 24 to 48 hours after the vasectomy. Also get an ice pack to use later. Before the surgery, use scissors to trim the hair around your penis and scrotum to about 1/4 inch, so this does not have to be done in the doctor's office. (You do not need to cut or shave the pubic hair above your testicles and penis.) Then shower or bathe to get rid of the loose hair and wash your testicles and penis thoroughly with soap.

Bring an athletic supporter or a snug pair of briefs with you to wear after the operation. (Briefs are likely to be softer and less irritating than a supporter.) This will hold the dressings in place and, by supporting the testicles, protect the incision area from strain and discomfort. Your physician can help you put on the supporter and briefs. Even after the incision or puncture no longer needs a bandage, you should continue to wear the support until you are completely healed.

If possible, schedule the operation for a Thursday or Friday so you will have the weekend for recuperation. The less active you are for a few days after the vasectomy, the lower your risk of having a complication.

After the Operation

Get the telephone number and name of the person to call if you have any questions at any time later on or if you experience unusual discomfort. Check with the physician or nurse about how often to change the dressing. Gauze pads can be bought at drugstores, or your vasectomist may provide you with a supply. Keep a bandage on the wound for as long as your doctor indicates.

Once at home, spend most of that day and the next with your feet up—literally. Periodically put the ice pack on your scrotum for the first day to reduced the chance that the incision area will swell or bleed. If necessary, take a non-aspirin, over-the-counter pain reliever such as acetaminophen. Check your choice of medication and the dosage with your physician before you leave the office or clinic.

Avoid strenous physical activity—any hard exertion that will strain or put pressure on your groin or scrotum.

It is normal to have some pain, swelling, and discoloration in the immediate area of the incision or puncture for a few days, or sometimes longer. This is less likely to occur, however, if you have had the no-scalpel procedure. A small amount of blood or clear fluid may ooze from the incision for a day or two. The gauze bandage will absorb this and protect the incision from being irritated by your clothes. If a single pad does not seem to be enough, use several. If these symptoms grow worse, get in touch with the practitioner who performed the vasectomy or with your regular physician.

AFTER-VASECTOMY DANGER SIGNS

Call your physician immediately if you experience any of these symptoms:

- Fever—a temperature over 100.4 degrees F—within a week after the operation.
- Swelling near the incision that is larger than a quarter, or pus or continual bleeding from the incision or puncture.
- Pain in the area of incision or in the scrotum that gets worse or does not go away in a day or two.

To keep the incision dry for the first couple of days, do not shower or take a bath or go swimming. When you do bathe or shower, wash the incision area gently but thoroughly.

In the rare instance that the sutures were not the absorbable type, you will need an appointment to have the stitches removed.

Sexual Intercourse

The rule for having intercourse after a vasectomy is to wait until it feels comfortable, anywhere from a few days to a week or two. If your scrotum is still sore, you can reduce the vigor of your lovemaking.

After the operation there is still stored-up sperm in the semen for some time, so you or your partner need to use some kind of birth control until at least two tests of your semen show no sperm are present. Do not skip these tests: most vasectomy failures show up (as pregnancies) in the first year afterwards.

Some men also have pain in the scrotum, as testicular fluid and sperm build up behind the surgical obstruction before being absorbed by the body. The chance of this occurring may be reduced by leaving the cut ends of the vas open. Regardless of which method is used, the congestion goes away after a few months.

COST

A vasectomy costs between $350 and $1,000, depending on where you live and who performs it. As a rule, this cost includes two or three postoperative visits for testing your semen for sperm. Sometimes this charge includes the first consultation, but often the first visit is billed separately, because a substantial number of men who have a consultation do not go on to have the surgery. Many health insurance plans, HMOs, and Medicaid pay for vasectomies.

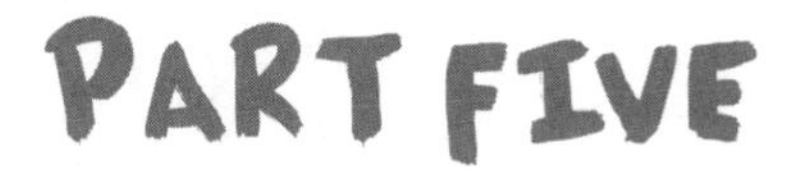

Other Methods of Fertility Control

14
Cycle-Based Fertility Awareness Methods

Cycle-based fertility awareness methods depend on an understanding of the fertile period in a woman's menstrual cycle and abstaining from sex during those days. These birth control methods are called "natural" by some people because women learn to interpret the normal physical signs of their bodies that signal the beginning and end of fertility each month. However, it is not necessarily natural for couples to avoid having intercourse for many days out of each month, which these methods require.

The rhythm, or calendar rhythm, method was the first of these to be used, and it is still the most common. Other approaches, however, such as the cervical mucus and symptothermal methods, give a woman a better understanding of her physiology and her fertility cycle and are more accurate. The use of calendar rhythm alone is not encouraged today because it leads to many unintended pregnancies.

All the fertility awareness methods are based on the fact that the probability of pregnancy is negligible except for about 10 days in the middle of a typical menstrual cycle. Although typical menstrual cycles may vary from 23 to 35 days in length, with even shorter and longer cycles possible, this "fertile phase" is almost always the same length. The key to the successful use of cycle-based birth control is learning when in the cycle the possible fertile days occur and refraining from sex (or using another form of contraception) during those days. If abstinence is the choice, this can mean avoiding intercourse for one-third to one-half of the month, possibly using other ways to achieve orgasm without intercourse.

Cycle-based methods today are known most often by two labels: natural family planning (NFP) and fertility awareness methods (FAM). Regardless of the label, the techniques used to determine a woman's fertile period are very similar. The difference lies in what is done with the information.

Natural family planning is generally learned within the context of religious beliefs about birth control, and the couples who practice it use abstinence during fertile days to avoid pregnancy. In contrast, couples who practice the fertility awareness method might have intercourse during the fertile days and use a barrier method to avert pregnancy. Fertility observation also can be used chiefly to improve the effectiveness of barrier methods. A woman and her partner can take extra precautions during those days, such as using extra spermicide in addition to a diaphragm or condom.

Fertility observation has the important advantages of having no negative side effects and costing very little. In addition, when pregnancy is desired, a woman's awareness of when she is fertile can be useful in helping her conceive.

The disadvantage of these methods is that, to be successful, they require real commitment and diligent practice. More training is needed for them than for other methods of contraception, because the signs of fertility can differ from cycle to cycle and from woman to woman. Couples who master the techniques of fertility awareness, however, and successfully integrate this knowledge into their sexual life can achieve very high rates of success.

The best source for classes in these methods is the Catholic Church, which offers them through "Marriage and Family Life" offices or programs run by local Catholic archdioceses. Classes generally are held once a month for 3 or 4 months and are open to any couple interested in a natural method of contraception, regardless of religious background, or lack of religious background. About

IN A NUTSHELL

FERTILITY AWARENESS METHODS

A woman uses these methods to recognize changes in her body that indicate the fertile phase of her menstrual cycle. If she does not want to get pregnant, she must not have sex during those days. Women who become very familiar with their body's changes can be successful in preventing pregnancy.

For these methods to work for you, your partner has to be willing to avoid sex during the many days in each month that it is possible to get pregnant. If you are not sure about your safe days or if you and your partner take chances, these methods have a high failure rate.

Classes that teach fertility awareness are available, usually through the Catholic Church.

Fertility awareness methods do not protect against STDs, including AIDS.

one-fourth of those who take such classes are not of the Catholic faith. Catholic hospitals also may offer classes or be able to provide information on local programs.

Like many of the other contraceptive methods, cycle-based birth control does not protect against the transmission of sexually transmitted diseases, including AIDS.

THE MENSTRUAL CYCLE

An understanding of what happens in the female body during the course of the menstrual cycle is helpful in appreciating how these techniques work. (Also see Chapter 1 on anatomy.)

The first day of menstruation is day one of the cycle. Menstruation takes place because an egg that was released from an ovary during the preceding weeks was not fertilized and did not implant in the blood-rich endometrium, the lining of the uterus. As a result, the uterus sloughs off the endometrium—and that is menstruation.

On the first day of menstruation, a new cycle begins as the pituitary gland releases follicle-stimulating hormone (FSH). As its name implies, FSH activates the follicles of the ovary to enlarge and the egg cells within them to grow. In addition, the follicles begin to secrete estrogen.

As the amount of estrogen in the body increases, the cervix begins to produce cervical mucus in steadily larger amounts. The cervical os (its opening) begins to widen as the mucus becomes abundant, watery, and stretchy. The wide open os and the plentiful, "fertile" mucus make it easier for sperm to move swiftly into the uterus and fallopian tubes—toward any egg cell that may be there. The type of mucus secreted at this time protects the sperm from the normal acidic vaginal secretions, which can kill sperm.

While the reproductive tract is becoming hospitable to sperm, the increased level of estrogen also stimulates the pituitary to secrete luteinizing hormone (LH). The resulting surge of LH triggers the release of a mature egg cell from its follicle, so it can be caught by the fimbria and guided into a fallopian tube.

The empty follicle begins to produce progesterone. This hormone stimulates the os to close and the cervical cells to stop making fertile mucus. In most women, it also causes the basal body temperature to rise several fractions of a degree. The temperature remains elevated until progesterone declines, the endometrium begins to be sloughed off, and the menstrual cycle begins again. If the egg has been fertilized and implants itself in the uterus, the endometrium stays in place in order to nurture the egg as it divides and grows, and menstruation does not occur.

A follicle releases an egg (ovulation) approximately 14 days before the onset of menstruation, regardless of the length of an individual woman's menstrual cycle. If the cervical mucus is hospitable, it is believed that sperm can survive in the reproductive tract for as long as 7 days. Eggs can live 12 to 24 hours. Sometimes a second egg is released a day or so after the first, making fraternal twins possible.

Allowing for inaccuracies in the timing of ovulation, even women with regular cycles must assume that they could become pregnant for up to 10 days during each cycle. A woman with an irregular menstrual cycle who wants to be safe from conception must consider her probable fertile period to be as long as 13 to 14 days. Long fertile phases can be a strain for couples who rely on abstinence for unsafe days, although many couples find ways other than vaginal intercourse to reach sexual satisfaction.

ARE YOU A GOOD CANDIDATE FOR CYCLE-BASED BIRTH CONTROL?

Fertility awareness methods of contraception work best for couples who are monogamous, because these methods require sharing the responsibility with a reliable sexual partner. A monogamous relationship is additionally important because these methods often involve unprotected intercourse and do not prevent sexually transmitted diseases.

Good candidates are couples who are strongly motivated not to have children and genuinely do not mind the organization and discipline needed to succeed. Couples who do not mind abstaining from intercourse and are comfortable reaching orgasm by other means also may find these methods suitable.

Men and women who dislike the interruption of certain contraceptives or worry about the side effects of hormonal methods may prefer to combine the fertility awareness approach with a barrier method for fertile days.

Women and men who for religious reasons choose not to use other methods of birth control are also good candidates for cycle-based family planning.

FERTILITY AWARENESS DEVICES

Ovulation predictor kits that are available in drugstores can detect ovulation only 24 to 48 hours beforehand, not soon enough to alert a couple to avoid intercourse, considering the survival ability of sperm. The kits are designed for couples who are trying to achieve pregnancy and cannot be used either to replace or enhance the fertility awareness methods described in this chapter.

EFFECTIVENESS

It is difficult to establish an accurate failure rate for cycle-based methods. They work better for couples who are older, have used them for a while, and are highly motivated. The most recent estimated failure rates for the first year of using cycle-based methods range from 1 to 25 percent. Among perfect users, first year failure rates have varied from 1 to 9 percent, depending on the individual method. Among the more typical users, however, 20 percent become pregnant during the first year.

Failure rates are lowest if couples limit unprotected sex strictly to the period *after* ovulation; failures are more common if unprotected sex occurs before ovulation.

Inadequate teaching, incomplete acceptance of this approach, a high dropout rate, and careless use of the technique are some of the reasons for the failure of cycle-based methods. For best results, it is important to find a health practitioner or family life instructor certified in these methods. They can be learned best from personal instruction, not from reading materials, because a couple may need assistance in changing their sexual attitudes and behaviors. Young women whose periods are just beginning and women who are approaching menopause particularly need skilled input in order to use fertility awareness methods.

CYCLE-BASED METHODS

Four main fertility awareness methods are practiced today. They can be used alone or, as often happens, can be combined to improve the rate of success. Variations of a particular method also may be taught in some places.

Calendar Rhythm Method

This method was the earliest technique used to establish the fertile and infertile days of a woman's menstrual cycle. It was devised in the 1930s, when it was determined that ovulation usually precedes menstruation by a predictable number of days (approximately 14) every month, regardless of the total length of the cycle. Figuring out the length of the fertile period had to take into account the number of days the egg was thought to be in the fallopian tubes, available to be fertilized, plus the number of days sperm could live in a woman's reproductive tract. This method uses a three-step formula.

Step 1. Make a calendar-like record of the beginning and end of at least eight menstrual cycles. The first day of bleeding, no matter how light, is day one of the cycle. The last day of the cycle is the day before the next menstrual period. After you chart your cycles in this fashion, note the number of days of the longest and the shortest cycles.

Step 2. To calculate the most likely first day of your fertile period, substract *18 days* from the number of days in your *shortest* menstrual cycle. If your shortest cycle was 24 days, subtracting 18 days indicates that day 6 of your cycle is the earliest probable time you could be fertile.

Step 3. To calculate the probable last day of the fertile period, subtract *11 days* from the number of days of the *longest* cycle. If your longest cycle was 33 days, for example, subtracting 11 days from 33 puts the last probable day of your fertile period at day 22.

To avoid pregnancy in this example, you would have to abstain from intercourse, or use a barrier contraceptive, from day 6 to day 22 of your cycle. Your safe period is from day 23, through your next menstrual period, through day 5 of your new cycle, including days 23 and 5. During such cycles, this schedule provides approximately 5 to 6 menstruation-free days per month for unprotected intercourse. Many women have irregular cycles, with the result that their potentially fertile periods, as figured by the calendar method, can be long and their safe periods short.

The best way to keep track of fertile and infertile days is to mark them off each month on a calendar. Even if you have established what your menstrual pattern is, continue to record your cycles by indicating the day each period begins. If your cycles begin to fluctuate considerably in length, so that you seem to have more fertile days than usual, get in touch with the instructor or health practitioner who has been helping you with this method.

Temperature Method

Basal body temperature (BBT) is your resting temperature. By charting your BBT for 3 or 4 months, you can determine when you usually ovulate. Just before ovulation, a woman's BBT typically drops a few fractions of a degree. After ovulation, the BBT usually rises between 0.4 and 0.8 degrees F and remains at that higher level every day until just before menstruation begins. What is important is not the temperature, but the fact that it rose over your normal baseline temperature. If you do not have such a sustained rise in your BBT, you may not have ovulated.

It is vital to take your basal body temperature in the morning before you get out of bed, talk, or take a drink of any fluid, hot or cold. You must also have had at least 3 hours of sleep to get an accurate reading. This means you also can record your BBT if you wake up in the middle of the night, as long as you have had 3 hours of sleep. You can take your temperature orally, rectally, or vaginally, but use the same method every time. Leave the thermometer in place for as long as its instructions dictate.

Special BBT thermometers, designed for reading fractional changes in temperature, cost approximately $12 and are available in drugstores. (They register only the temperature range between 90 degrees and 100 degrees F.) To use the thermometer, shake it down to 96 degrees and put it next to your bed the evening before. If you use it rectally, lubricate the bulb. Monthly charts for noting each day's BBT are available from your doctor or your family planning clinic, or you can make your own.

A change in the BBT of only a fraction of a degree is important. Mark each tenth of a degree with a dot on your chart. Connecting the dots makes it easy to see the day-to-day changes. After you have charted each day's temperature for several months, you will begin to see a pattern. Your temperature changes may be steep, gradual, or in steps. Your chart may contain some unexpected blips that represent a sleepless night or an emotional upset, but that does not affect the overall pattern. If there are unusual high or low readings any morning and you can figure out the cause, make a note on the chart to help you interpret the readings later on.

You should see a pattern of 1 to 3 low-temperature days before ovulation—the highly fertile days—and then a progesterone-caused rise in temperature. After 3 days of higher temperature you are safely infertile. Because the temperature rise is triggered by progesterone produced *after* ovulation, this method cannot be used as an advance warning of ovulation. It is an indication, however, that ovulation has taken place and the fertile period is about to end.

The safest way to use the BBT method is to abstain from intercourse or use a barrier method through the first half of your cycle.

There are several events other than ovulation that can cause a rise in BBT. They include:

- Illness accompanied by a fever can cause variations in your current cycle and in the next one. A low-grade infection, cold, or flu can cause a rise of a few tenths of a degree, enough to affect the BBT.
- Alcoholic drinks in the evening may cause a rise in the BBT the next morning in some women.
- Taking your BBT later than usual may result in a higher reading. If this happens, record the time difference on your chart.

Cervical Mucus Method

The technique commonly used today by women to recognize the variations in their cervical mucus was developed in the 1970s by Drs. John and Evelyn Billings. A more standardized version is widely taught in the United States as the Creighton model.

The mucus method is useful for determining when *before ovulation* it may be possible to have unprotected sex without conceiving. Recognizable changes in mucus can signal the onset of the fertile period more clearly than does the BBT. *After ovulation*, however, the basal body temperature may be a more accurate way of knowing when your infertile period has begun and you can have unprotected sex.

The secretions from the cervix change during the course of each month. The days immediately following menstruation are called the "dry" days, when the cervix secretes very little mucus. These days are considered fairly safe for unprotected intercourse because ovulation is unlikely, and there is no mucus to help sperm survive the naturally acid environment of the vagina. (Some women do not have dry days, especially if they have very short cycles.)

After the few dry days, the mucus is still skimpy, but becomes sticky to the touch, does not stretch, and appears somewhat white, yellow, or cloudy. (Appearance can vary from woman to woman.) This mucus usually is a sign that the estrogen levels are rising. When this type of mucus is present, egg development has begun and unprotected intercourse is no longer safe.

A few days just before actual ovulation, the body's high estrogen levels cause the mucus to become much more abundant. It now looks clear and feels thin, slippery, and very stretchy and has the consistency of raw egg white. Some women can take a bit of it and stretch it between thumb and forefinger into a thin strand of 2 to 3 inches or more. This stretchability is called *spinnbarkeit* and is characteristic of this time of the cycle. Spinnbarkeit mucus is also called fertile-type mucus because it helps sperm to survive and reach the egg. Its presence is a sign that ovulation is about to take place. Many women are aware of this mucus as a wet feeling at the mouth of the vagina.

The estrogen spurt that triggers the production of fertile-type mucus typically begins several days before ovulation. The last day that this type of mucus can be felt is the day of peak fertility, when the ovary releases an egg. However, the only definite way to know that peak fertility and ovulation have occurred is 3 or 4 days afterward, when the mucus is definitely back to being sticky and skimpy.

From the fourth day after the peak day until the end of the monthly cycle, when you menstruate again, you are infertile. During this infertile phase, you usually will have little mucus for 7 to 12 days. A few days before your period begins, however, it may become a bit more abundant.

This description of the cervical mucus cycle may be true for many women, but not for all. You will not be able to use this method effectively until you understand your individual pattern. For the first month, you must record your mucus quality every day. And you must note the days when there is no mucus. Many women can see their pattern after one month, while others need more time and help from their health care provider or family planning instructor. Many fertility awareness counselors suggest complete abstinence from sex during the first cycle being charted, in order to avoid confusing the mucus with semen or normal sexual lubrication. With

LATE OVULATION

Ovulation can be delayed if anxiety, stress, illness, or a change in your life occurs after your last menstrual period and before ovulation. If you then have a peak day that does not seem normal, during the following three days carefully check the characteristics of your mucus. Fertile mucus may reappear, indicating that ovulation was delayed and now at last is taking place. If it is not clear that the peak occurred and the infertile period started, postpone sex or use a barrier method.

experience, most women learn to tell the difference between these secretions.

When using this method, remember that douching is likely to wash out any mucus and a lubricant or spermicidal jelly could be confused with mucus. If you have a discharge from an infection, postpone mucus charting until it is cleared up. When you begin keeping a record, touch the mouth of your vagina every day to check for mucus and make a brief note of what you find—what it feels and looks like and whether it is skimpy or abundant. Also write down any other physical signs that may indicate a change in your fertility cycle.

During the infertile phase, the cervix is lower in the vagina and easier to reach. It feels firm to the touch and the os is closed. As ovulation approaches, the cervix withdraws higher in the vaginal canal and feels broader and softer. The os also begins to dilate so that you can actually feel the opening. Look for and record these changes. Other signs of ovulation are a pain on either side of the abdomen (known as *mittelschmerz*), breast tenderness, feelings of heaviness, or abdominal swelling. After ovulation, the cervix is again low in the vagina and feels firm and closed. Even though you may have no mucus at all at this time, you should be able to detect the other cervical changes that offer clues to your fertility pattern.

Although the mucus method alone can be an adequate guide, some health care practitioners recommend that it be combined with the temperature method for greater effectiveness. A great deal depends on the clarity of your record of mucus changes and on your

COUPLES WHO ARE NOT GOOD CANDIDATES FOR THESE METHODS

Women who absolutely must not get pregnant because of serious medical problems that would be worsened by pregnancy—and who would not have an abortion—are not good candidates. They are better served by a contraceptive that has an extremely reliable high rate of effectiveness.

Couples who find it difficult to refrain from vaginal intercourse for a number of days also are not good candidates, especially if they do not use barrier methods. Finally, women who are poor sleepers or travel a great deal cannot use the temperature method effectively, because lack of sleep and jet lag can affect the BBT.

temperature charts. When several months of experience with both methods demonstrate that the cervical mucus method is an accurate indicator of ovulation, you may feel comfortable using it alone.

The mucus method alone sometimes has uncertainties. As we mentioned, it can be difficult to distinguish between cervical mucus and normal vaginal secretions or a discharge caused by a vaginal infection. And it takes some practice to be able to tell the difference between mucus and vaginal medications, semen, or the lubrication that follows sexual arousal.

The mucus method does have several advantages over the other fertility awareness techniques. It does not require taking the basal body temperature every day. For women with very irregular periods, it requires fewer days of abstinence. And it is more effective than the calendar rhythm method.

Symptothermal Method

Because using any one method of fertility awareness alone may not be foolproof, many counselors recommend the symptothermal method, which combines checking your cervical mucus, recording your BBT, and watching for the other signs of ovulation. The symptothermal approach is particularly useful if you tend to have unusually long or short cycles, because the combination of methods helps to pinpoint your fertile phase.

You can record your BBT, mucus, and calendar information on the same chart. When using the symptothermal method, it is important to remember that the safe, infertile period begins: after 3 days of a consistent rise in BBT; after 3 days of having a closed, firm, low cervix; and on the fourth day after the peak mucus day. Both the *mucus change* and the *temperature rise* must occur before unprotected intercourse can be resumed safely. Changes in the cervix are used only to verify the other events.

It is a good idea to record the onset of your period, your daily BBT, your type of mucus, and your other signs until you are certain you know when you ovulate. From that point you can use only one method, if you wish.

FINDING A FERTILITY AWARENESS CLASS

Since cycle-based birth control methods (especially when combined with abstinence) can be difficult regimens to follow at first, it is strongly recommended that couples—or women—join support groups, women's health networks, or family life programs that offer classes in such methods. Personal feedback and support from other users of these methods are very helpful, especially during your first months of learning about cycles. Many churches and church-run hospitals offer family life programs and support groups. You need not be a church member to participate.

In many cities, the Catholic archdiocese has family life programs that teach natural family planning. A parish priest or teachers in local Catholic schools may be helpful in finding the nearest family life program. Many Planned Parenthood clinics or women's health centers also may have someone who is certified to teach the cycle-based methods.

Church-sponsored programs discourage the use of barrier contraceptives during fertile days but are good sources of education in the basics of natural methods. Your decision to use a condom, diaphragm, or cervical cap can be a private one. If your local women's health center or Planned Parenthood clinic teaches cycle-based methods, it is most likely to teach fertility awareness plus the use of any barrier method you choose.

If you have no local source on how to find instruction in cycle-based methods, you can write the Natural Family Planning Program, National Conference of Catholic Bishops, 3211 Fourth St. N.E., Washington, D.C., 20017, for information on the classes nearest you. The Program's telephone is 202-541-3240; its fax number is 202-541-3203.

Remember that it is important to find a teacher who has been certified by a school of natural family planning. Much of the effectiveness of these methods depends on how competently they are taught.

COST

Cycle-based methods are inexpensive. There may be a small fee for the classes and you may need to buy record-keeping charts and a thermometer if you use the temperature or symptothermal method.

15

Withdrawal

Withdrawal is a method of birth control that requires a man to remove his penis from the vagina when he feels he is about to ejaculate. Ejaculation then takes place outside the woman's body, completely away from her vaginal area, to protect her from any contact with his sperm. Withdrawal costs nothing, is always available, and does not require using any devices or chemical-based products. Although it causes no side effects, withdrawal can interrupt intercourse at its climax, or before, and may markedly decrease both partners' sexual pleasure. Because it can have a high failure rate, it may be more acceptable to couples who are interested in spacing—rather than preventing—births.

Men who cannot control their orgasms and men who have premature ejaculations are not very successful in using this method for contraception. Men who use withdrawal need very good control and an awareness of exactly when they are about to ejaculate. It is difficult for a man to remove his penis from the vagina just when his instincts tell him to penetrate further. If he starts withdrawing too late, he may leave some semen at the opening of the vagina, making it possible for sperm to move up into the reproductive tract.

Needless to say, women may not be enthusiastic about this

method. It is not easy for a woman to relax completely and reach an orgasm when she is wondering whether her partner will be able to pull out in time or whether he will have to withdraw his penis before she has reached a full sexual response, bringing a sudden, uncomfortable end to lovemaking. It also puts the man completely in control of the sex act and of contraception, unless the couple uses one of the control techniques described below that help men control arousal and postpone ejaculation.

On the other hand, couples who have been together long enough to understand each other's sexual rhythms may be able to achieve satisfactory sexual responses when using withdrawal.

Withdrawal provides no protection against sexually transmitted diseases, including AIDS.

EFFECTIVENESS

Calculating the effectiveness of the withdrawal method is difficult. Only 2 percent of couples in the United States use this method. In a 1990 analysis, the lowest failure rate was 4 percent in the first year when withdrawal was reported to be used perfectly. More typical users had a failure rate of 19 percent during the first year.

USING WITHDRAWAL

Couples who communicate well and can be cooperative in their lovemaking are more likely to be successful in using this method. Moreover, control techniques do exist (see below), such as the "squeeze" technique and the "stop-start" method, that can make withdrawal more effective and more pleasurable for both partners.

In practicing withdrawal, before the penis is inserted the tip should be carefully wiped off to remove any pre-ejaculate fluid. Although it is not known whether pre-ejaculate carries many sperm, to be on the safe side any fluid should be removed. You may wish to keep a box of tissues handy for this purpose, for cleaning up ejaculate and, perhaps, for ejaculating into.

A backup spermicide could be somewhat useful in case semen accidently spills into the vaginal opening or vagina. Adding spermicide afterward may futile, however, because sperm move so rapidly. Douching definitely is not helpful and may actually speed sperm on their way.

IN A NUTSHELL

WITHDRAWAL

This is a method used by a man in which he withdraws his penis from the woman when he feels he is going to come (ejaculate). He then ejaculates outside her body. There are a couple of techniques that make this method easier, but withdrawal requires great control and much practice. It also decreases sexual pleasure for both partners.

Withdrawal costs nothing and is always available, but it has a high failure rate. It is used mostly by married couples who want to space their children.

Withdrawal does not protect against disease. A condom plus a spermicide are the best safeguards against STDs and AIDS for sexually active people.

Control Techniques

Two exercises have been practiced successfully for many years to help men control their sexual excitement and postpone ejaculation. Both exercises—the "squeeze" and the "stop-start"—require the willingness and cooperation of both partners. Used regularly, the exercises can be quite successful.

The Squeeze Technique. The penis squeeze technique has been employed for many years by Masters and Johnson and other sex therapists to help men overcome a tendency toward premature ejaculation. It can be a very helpful exercise for couples who wish to practice withdrawal, because it gives the man greater control over the timing of his orgasm, thus prolonging the sexual pleasure of each partner and increasing the efficacy of this method.

The couple may stroke and caress each other's genitals, including the penis, without penetration taking place, up to the time when the man senses he is about to ejaculate. He signals this to his partner, who immediately takes the penis in her hand, placing her thumb just underneath the tip (the glans), with her forefinger and middle finger across the top of the glans—one finger on each side of the bump (the coronal ridge). If the man is uncircumcised, the woman can feel the coronal ridge through the foreskin covering the glans, but the place underneath the glans where she should press her thumb may have to be located by guesswork.

When the penis is erect, squeezing it firmly usually causes no discomfort, although this is not true for every man. This should halt his immediate urge to ejaculate, yet have only a slight softening effect on the erection. Because the response to such pressure is individual, couples may wish to experiment to determine just how much pressure is necessary to be effective. With her fingers in the position described, the woman exerts as much pressure as needed for 4 or 5 seconds. (Some women may have to use both hands to be effective.)

When the man feels his impulse to ejaculate has worn off sufficiently, which may take anywhere from a few seconds to a few minutes, sexual stimulation can be resumed, with the expectation that the urge to ejaculate will be postponed for about 10 to 20 minutes.

When the man has developed a certain amount of control over his ejaculation, it is then possible for the couple to go a step further, to vaginal penetration combined with the squeeze technique, to prolong intercourse. They may use the spoon position or the woman may place herself above the man. When he is about to ejaculate, he warns her, and she immediately removes his penis from her vagina and uses the squeeze technique to stop his orgasm. This approach is safe as long as the man lets his partner know when an orgasm is imminent. Obviously, it is important that he not wait until the very last minute, when it is too late for the squeeze to work.

The Stop-Start Method. Instead of—or in addition to—the squeeze technique, ejaculation can be delayed and intercourse prolonged by the stop-start or stop-and-go method. This means intercourse is prolonged by completely stopping all sexual stimulation, including thrusting with the penis, as soon as ejaculation becomes imminent. After about 30 seconds of quietness, the intense desire to ejaculate begins to ebb. When the urge has noticeably subsided, lovemaking is resumed.

Both of these exercises require practice before they feel easy and natural. As the techniques are repeated, the man becomes accustomed to receiving prolonged pleasure from sexual stimulation. He

achieves greater mastery over his ejaculation and becomes able to postpone his orgasms for long periods.

As a couple uses these exercises to help the man develop more control of his sexual performance, the woman may also have to find when she is most stimulated to having an orgasm. In the beginning, it may be safer for her to have her orgasm before or after her partner approaches his climax, so she can assist in the withdrawal technique. As he gains more control over his arousal so that sexual stimulation for both of them can be drawn out, the woman may have more time in which to reach her climax. With practice, each partner may be able to experience more than one orgasm and still practice withdrawal effectively.

The Spoon Position

The spoon position makes it easier for both partners to exert some control over the man's ejaculation and for him to withdraw. The man and woman curl up together on their sides, with the man behind the woman. This position allows him to hold her closely and to caress her, while at the same time the angle of their bodies makes it impossible for his penis to penetrate too deeply into her vagina.

The spoon position is comfortable for the woman and permits her to stroke her partner's penis and to enjoy his stimulation of her breasts and clitoris. Her legs are together rather than apart, which also helps control the deepness of her partner's thrust.

16

Emergency Contraception

No contraceptive works perfectly. Condoms break, you can forget to use your spermicide, diaphragms and cervical caps move out of place. Women sometimes are forced to have sex, and couples have sex unexpectedly without protecting themselves against pregnancy.

If the unprotected intercourse was a single event and you act quickly, emergency contraception can help prevent pregnancy. It is neither complicated nor expensive—and it is safe, legal, and usually readily available. Two methods of emergency contraception are available in the United States. One is a short course (two times in one day) of a higher dose of ordinary birth control pills. Treatment should be started within 72 hours after sex took place. It prevents pregnancy about 75 percent of the time. The pill used is not an abortion pill. The second method is the insertion of the copper IUD (the ParaGard).

Although using emergency contraception obviously is critical only if your cycle is in its fertile phase at the time you had unprotected intercourse, if you are not positive about where you are in your cycle, it is better to be safe than sorry. Because the treatment is both safe and available, use it if you are in any doubt about the possibility of pregnancy.

EMERGENCY CONTRACEPTION HOTLINE

FOR INFORMATION ABOUT TREATMENT METHODS AND HOW TO FIND A HEALTH CARE PRACTITIONER NEAR YOU WHO PROVIDES EMERGENCY CONTRACEPTION, CALL THE NATIONAL HOTLINE: 1-888-NOT-2-LATE

(This hotline is operated by the Reproductive Health Technologies Project.)

NOTE: The use of emergency contraception does not cause an induced abortion. It *prevents* an unintended pregnancy and thus reduces the need for an abortion.

Medical science defines the beginning of a pregnancy as the implantation of a fertilized egg in the lining of the uterus. Implantation takes place 5 to 7 days after an egg is fertilized. Emergency contraceptives work before implantation, not afterward.

TWO METHODS

Using Combined Pills or Minipills

The effectiveness of this treatment is time dependent. If more than 72 hours pass before you seek emergency contraception, the fertilized egg may have already reached the uterus and begun to implant itself. Emergency contraception needs to go to work *before* the fertilized egg implants in the uterus.

Combined Pills. Any of several brands of birth control pills that combine estrogen and progestin can be used. Depending on the brand, you either take two, four, or five combined pills, followed by two, four, or five pills 12 hours later. These should be started within 72 hours of the unprotected intercourse. The total amount of hormone is moderate, yet it is sufficient to have an effect: to inhibit ovulation, to slow the passage of the fertilized egg so it reaches the uterus at the wrong time, or to alter the lining of the uterus, which prevents the implanting of a fertilized egg. (For more information on the Pill, see Chapter 7.)

The standard emergency contraception is the Yuzpe method, which uses a birth control pill called "Ovral." Taking two Ovral as soon as possible within 72 hours after the unprotected intercourse and two additional Ovral 12 hours after the first dose adds up to a total of 200 micrograms of estrogen (ethinyl estradiol) and 2 milligrams of progestin (norgestrel). This regimen is very safe—there are no known reasons for not using it.

Minipills. The progestin-only pills that have been tested for this use are those containing levonorgestrel. You will need to take 20 of these pills within 48 hours after unprotected sex and a second dose of 20 more pills 12 hours later. These minipills seem to be as effective as combined birth control pills for this purpose, but are less likely to cause nausea and vomiting and other side effects (see Chapter 8.)

IN A NUTSHELL

EMERGENCY CONTRACEPTION

Emergency contraception means using a copper IUD or birth control pills to prevent pregnancy after unprotected intercourse. If pills are used within 72 hours after unprotected sex has taken place, they prevent about 75 percent of the pregnancies that would have occurred. An IUD can be effective if it is inserted up to 7 days after unprotected sex.

The emergency method used most often is a double dose of one of the stronger combined contraceptive pills. Twelve hours later, another double dose is taken.

Emergency contraception is not the same as a medical abortion. Emergency contraception prevents pregnancy.

Emergency contraception is prescribed by a doctor or clinic nurse after unprotected sex or an accident with a birth control method. It is also used after a rape.

Emergency contraception does not protect against STDs.

You can get toll-free information about this method by calling 1-888-NOT-2-LATE.

Using a Copper IUD

If you choose to have an IUD inserted instead, it can be put in place up to 7 days after the unprotected intercourse in order to prevent pregnancy. This method, however, should be chosen only if you want to continue to use it as a contraceptive. (For more information on IUDs, see Chapter 11.) The ParaGard can be left in place to provide continuous and very effective contraception for up to 10 years.

IUDs are not ideal for all women, however. Women at risk for sexually transmitted diseases because they or their partners have other sexual partners are not good candidates for IUDs. Insertion while an infection is present can lead to pelvic inflammatory disease, which can cause infertility if not noticed and treated. Because of this concern, women who have been raped are not good candidates for emergency insertion of an IUD. However, the risk of pelvic infection from an IUD insertion is small among women in long-term, mutually monogamous relationships who are at little risk for STDs.

The copper IUD alters the endometrium by causing an inflammatory reaction that makes the endometrium inhospitable to implantation by the egg. It also interferes with the fertilization and movement of the egg in the fallopian tubes.

EFFECTIVENESS

A regimen using the combined oral contraceptive Ovral was developed by Canadian physician Albert Yuzpe in the mid-1970s and tested on 1,300 Canadian women. Almost all the women began a menstrual period within 21 days of treatment.

Minipills and combined oral contraceptives reduce the chance of pregnancy by about 75 percent. This does not mean that 25 percent of women will become pregnant. If 100 women have unprotected sex once during the second or third week of their menstrual cycles (when a woman is most fertile), about eight will become pregnant. If those same 100 women had used the Pill or minipill treatment for emergency contraception, only two would have become pregnant, a 75 percent reduction. The efficacy of the treatment may be affected

USING PILLS FOR EMERGENCY CONTRACEPTION

Brand Name	Number of Pills to Take: As soon as possible	Number of Pills to Take: 12 hours later
Ovral	2	2
Lo/Ovral	4	4
Nordette	4	4
Levlen	4	4
Triphasil (yellow only)	4	4
Tri-Levlen (yellow only)	4	4
Alesse	5	5
Ovrette	20*	20

*Must be taken within 48 hours of unprotected intercourse (a progestin -only pill)

by the same medications that reduce the effect of birth control pills (see Chapter 7).

Emergency insertion of a copper IUD is 99 percent effective. If 1,000 women had unprotected sex once during their fertile days, an average of 80 would get pregnant. If they had had a copper IUD inserted, at most only one would become pregnant.

HEALTH EFFECTS

The side effects associated with emergency contraception are similar to those associated with the respective methods. For example, with a combined pill treatment you may experience some nausea (sometimes associated with vomiting) and breast tenderness. Some physicians and clinics automatically provide an antinausea medication to use in case of vomiting. Extra contraceptive pills are usually provided in case the first pills are vomited in the first hour. Some women may also experience abdominal pain, headache, or dizziness with this treatment, but all side effects usually subside quickly.

The progestin-only pill is less likely to produce such side effects. The possible side effects of having an IUD inserted are described above and in Chapter 11.

Emergency contraceptive pills may change the timing of your next menstrual period so that it is a few days earlier or later. If bleeding does not start within 3 weeks after the treatment, however, you should have a pregnancy test.

Another health issue associated with emergency contraception is the possible effect on the fetus if the treatment does not succeed and you become pregnant and decide to have the baby. Studies have found no increased risk of birth defects in cases where women continued to take birth control pills after they unknowingly were pregnant. Failure of the IUD method is extremely rare, but if it occurs, the IUD is removed and there is no known increased risk of birth defects.

USING EMERGENCY CONTRACEPTION

If you decide you need emergency contraception, obviously it is important to act swiftly. Although it is steadily becoming more available, in some parts of the United States it may take a little time to locate a provider.

Finding a Clinic or Practitioner

If your own doctor is not familiar with emergency contraception or unwilling to prescribe it, many women's health centers and family planning clinics, including Planned Parenthood clinics, offer emergency contraception. (Although many family physicians and gynecologists may be aware of this treatment, they may not be accustomed to providing it.) Doctors and nurse practitioners can provide this care. University and college health centers also may offer this service. If you are not a student, the centers may able to give you information or a referral.

Because this treatment is successful only if started very soon after unprotected intercourse, it is important to find assistance immediately.

When you telephone a practitioner or clinic, be prepared to answer the following questions:

- What was the date of your last menstrual period?
- Was it a normal period?
- On what date and at what time did the unprotected intercourse occur?
- Have you had unprotected intercourse at any other time since your last period?

Telephone screening saves vital time in scheduling you for emergency contraception or when referring you to another source of care, which sometimes is necessary. If you have serious health problems, for example, you almost always will be told to see a private physician for emergency contraception. If you call a clinic or practitioner because you were raped, you will probably be referred to the nearest rape crisis center or the emergency room of the local hospital. Rape is a criminal act, and rape centers are trained to gather evidence and deal with the other legal issues involved, as well as provide medical care and emotional counseling.

You should be aware that some antiabortion groups advertise in the Yellow Pages as "family planning centers" or abortion providers. They may discourage you from using emergency contraception. It can be difficult to tell the difference; however, if they will not set up an appointment for that day, they may not be a real health clinic. If they sound at all reluctant to see you promptly, ask why. If you are a candidate for emergency contraception, a legitimate clinic will schedule you to be seen right away or, if its schedule is too crowded, it will refer you to another source of care.

NOTE: If you do not have ready access to a health clinic that offers this treatment, you can call the emergency contraception hotline (1-888-not-2-late) for the name of clinicians in your area who provide emergency contraceptives.

The hotline will provide information on the methods and give you the names and telephone numbers of three health care practitioners in your area who provide this care. The hotline is accessible from any touch-tone telephone. If you live in an area where there are few providers, the nearest one may be several hours away, but you will still receive the names, locations, and telephone numbers of three practitioners.

EMERGENCY CONTRACEPTION TREATMENT

If you already are a patient of a particular health care provider or clinic and you have had a recent checkup, it may be possible to have the pills prescribed over the telephone.

If the practitioner you call does not know you or have your medical record, you will need to be scheduled for an emergency visit. You should be seen as soon as possible; if this cannot be done, find another provider right away.

If you are not a regular patient of the doctor or the clinic, a health history and a physical examination may be part of emergency contraception. You also will be asked to read and sign a simple informed consent form. Along with the contraceptive pills, you will be given an emergency telephone number to call if you experience any side effects. If an emergency number is not supplied, ask for it.

You will be given the pills and will probably be told to take the first ones at the clinic. The sooner the hormones enter your blood stream, the more effective they will be. You take the second set 12 hours after the first. You may want to time the first set of pills so that you do not have to wake up in the middle of the night to take the second set. (For example, if it is still within the 72 hour period, take them at 7 p.m. instead of 3 p.m.) Even if you become nauseated, the symptoms usually are very mild and disappear by the next day. (Some physicians suggest having a snack with the pills.)

If you vomit within 60 minutes of taking the pills, however, use the antinausea medication supplied by the clinic and then take the extra pills you were given. Follow them with the final set of pills 12 hours later. (If the practitioner is using Ovral, the most common method, you will take two pills.)

EMERGENCY CONTRACEPTION FOLLOWING RAPE

If you have been the victim of a sexual assault, seek care immediately. The best care is almost always found at a Rape Crisis Center, because you will need expert counseling, you may have been exposed to an STD and need to be tested and treated, and rape is a criminal act that should be reported to the police.

You can locate a Rape Crisis Center by calling the nearest hospital, a women's health center, or your local police or health department. If there is no such center in your community, the emergency room of the local hospital may have health care workers trained to handle this sort of emergency. If none is available, seek care at a family planning clinic, women's health center, or sympathetic private physician. Or call the Planned Parenthood clinic in the nearest large city for assistance.

At a Rape Crisis Center, you will be given a physical examination. Information is gathered on the sex acts performed, whether ejaculation took place, what sort of contraception you are using, and where you are in your menstrual cycle. A pregnancy test is performed to rule out the possibility of an earlier, unknown pregnancy. If you are not pregnant but are at risk for pregnancy from the rape, you will be treated with combined oral contraceptives to avert a pregnancy.

(If you do not get your next period after the rape, arrange for a pregnancy test. Many Rape Crisis Centers or Planned Parenthood clinics offer such tests if you do not have a physician of your own.)

A health care provider also will take blood and vaginal samples to test for gonorrhea, chlamydia, and syphilis. You will be given antibiotics to protect you against these STDs. You will also be counseled on how to deal with the possibility that you may have been infected with herpes or AIDS.

As part of the physical examination, evidence of the assault is collected. It is sent to the police crime laboratory and filed in case the rapist is caught and you want to have him prosecuted. In most cases, the evidence is labeled by number rather than name, in order to protect your privacy.

You may find it useful to discuss emergency contraception with your doctor or clinic before you need it. Practitioners are increasingly comfortable giving women a dose or two of emergency contraception in advance so they have it on hand just in case. And if your physician does not wish to provide emergency contraception, it is a good idea to locate a clinic or practitioner who will.

Emergency contraception is meant only for very occasional use and should not be considered a substitute for regular birth control. Regular birth control methods are much more effective and are less likely to cause nausea. If you need emergency contraception more than once or twice because your contraceptive method failed, you may want to consider changing methods.

COST

The cost of emergency contraception depends on what method you use and where you receive it. The cost for oral contraceptive treatment averages $60 for the office visit and the pills. If a pregnancy test is required, the cost is higher. If you want to be treated with minipills, the cost will be about $80 because two packs of Ovrette are needed. Most expensive is the emergency insertion of an IUD, which can range from $300 to $700 and includes the device itself, counseling, a physical exam, any necessary tests, and the insertion. Although this initial cost is high, the ParaGard IUD provides extremely effective contraception for at least 10 years.

Some clinics subsidize these costs for low-income women through sliding fees. Some insurance plans pay for emergency contraception. HMOs charge their usual low co-payments for office visits, prescriptions, and IUD insertion.

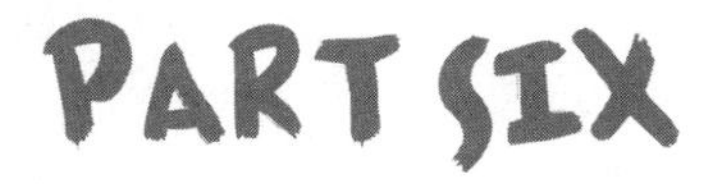

Other Issues of Birth Control

17

Breastfeeding and Contraception

Your contraceptive needs often change when you have a child. You may now feel your family is complete, or you simply may want to postpone your next pregnancy because you do not want to have children too close together.

Furthermore, if you wish to breastfeed, you need to know what birth control choices are appropriate and what influence contraceptives might have on the quality and quantity of breast milk. If you want a reliable contraceptive, there are methods that are both effective and compatible with breastfeeding. Most of all, you should be aware that exclusive breastfeeding can be very effective birth control in itself.

Breastfeeding, or lactation, delays your body's return to its usual cycle of ovulation. This also means you do not menstruate, because your uterus does not prepare for a fertilized egg. *Mothers who do not nurse* generally resume ovulation (and menstruation) within the first 3 months after their delivery. *For mothers who do breastfeed*, however, ovulation can be delayed for many months, sometimes as long as a year, depending on how often they nurse their babies. In the United States, the average delay in ovulation seldom lasts more than 6 months, because most mothers begin giving supplemental feedings, such as juice or cereal, by that time.

USING THE LACTATIONAL AMENORRHEA METHOD FOR BIRTH CONTROL

The absence of menstruation because of breastfeeding is called *lactational amenorrhea.* When used deliberately to prevent pregnancy, it is referred to as the lactational amenorrhea method (LAM). LAM can be continued for some months after a birth and used as a natural—and very effective—method of contraception. If you only breastfeed your baby, have no signs of menstruation, and have not passed the six-month postpartum mark, your risk of pregnancy while relying on lactational amenorrhea is less than 2 percent.

LAM can be maintained by following simple rules:

1. The intervals between nursing should not be longer than 4 hours. Working women who want to use LAM for birth control will need to pump their breasts at least every 4 hours while away from their babies.
2. Most of the baby's nutrition should come from breastfeeding. There should be little or no other foods or liquids given.
3. Six months should not have passed since your baby was born. (Using LAM beyond 6 months currently is not recommended.)
4. You have had no vaginal bleeding since the first month after your child was born.

How long menstruation is delayed depends a great deal on how completely you breastfeed. As long as your baby is suckling at least every 4 hours, ovulation usually will be suppressed. Either suckling or the stimulation of the nipple while using the breast pump inhibits the production of the hormone that is necessary for the ovaries to function. Without it, there is no ovulation and no menstrual cycle.

When you begin to supplement your infant's diet with other foods or liquids, nursing will become less frequent, and ovulation will soon get under way. *Any* vaginal bleeding (beyond the first 4 weeks following childbirth) means lactational amenorrhea has ended, and you need another contraceptive. Many women begin using birth control as soon as they start giving supplemental foods, before they

IN A NUTSHELL

BREASTFEEDING AND CONTRACEPTION

Breastfeeding can protect a woman against pregnancy for about 6 months after childbirth, if the baby is given no other food or milk and nurses often.

When you start giving your baby other food or milk, or if your periods begin, you must use birth control right away if you want to avoid another pregnancy.

If you want to use a contraceptive method while breastfeeding, some birth control methods are better than others. Good methods to use are condoms, diaphragms, the cervical cap, the IUD, and spermicides. If you have been using a diaphragm or cervical cap, you need to be refitted. The shape and size of your vagina and cervix may have changed.

Combined birth control pills are not recommended because the estrogen in the pills will decrease your milk supply. POPs may be used if you prefer pills to the methods above.

actually have any bleeding—because there is a risk that a fertile first ovulation will occur before any sign of menstruation.

It is a good idea to begin thinking about contraceptive methods before you actually need to use something. Since many couples resume sexual intercourse within weeks after childbirth, a woman who is not nursing or is only partially nursing should use birth control. If you are fully nursing, you will not need a contraceptive, but you should start planning which method will be best when you are no longer using LAM.

CONTRACEPTIVE METHODS FOR THE NURSING MOTHER

Although some women return to the birth control method they were using before they became pregnant, many others decide they need a more effective method or one more compatible with nursing. Many methods can be used safely when you have just given birth or are breastfeeding, but some are better than others.

Condoms pose no risk to either mother or child and offer protection against disease. Because a nursing mother's vagina is drier than normal, the use of a lubricated condom, a condom plus a spermicide, or a female condom will make this method more comfortable.

Whether or not you are breastfeeding, it is necessary to wait until the uterus has returned to its normal size and place and the cervix has closed before you are fitted for a *diaphragm* or *cervical cap*. If you have used either of these previously, you will need to be refitted, because the shape and size of your cervix and upper vagina may have changed.

Spermicides have not been shown to have an effect on breastfeeding, even though extremely small amounts of nonoxynol-9 may be absorbed into your bloodstream. Since vaginal dryness is common during nursing, some women find that spermicides, used alone or with a barrier contraceptive, make intercourse more comfortable.

IUDs are very suitable for nursing women, because they are convenient, effective, and safe. Neither the progesterone released from the Progestasert nor the copper of the ParaGard affects breast milk or the baby. The risk of the IUD being expelled by the uterus is reduced if it is inserted after the uterus has returned to normal size, about 6 weeks after the birth. There seems to be less discomfort when IUD insertion takes place during the breastfeeding months.

WHAT IS EXCLUSIVE BREASTFEEDING?

If you wish to use breastfeeding as a means of birth control, you must be nursing exclusively or almost exclusively, which is:

- nursing frequently, whenever the baby is hungry, both day and night;
- not offering the baby a bottle, pacifier, or other nipple substitute; and
- not supplementing breast milk with other sources of nourishment, such as juice or cow's milk.

When any of these criteria is not being met, it means that you are no longer exclusively (or almost exclusively) breastfeeding, and you cannot rely on LAM for birth control. When you start to give your baby other foods, or have to stop nursing for some reason (and do not want another child right away) you will need to start using some other form of contraception. Furthermore, any vaginal bleeding after the first month postpartum is also an indication that you should begin to use another method.

If you want this baby to be your last child, and have arranged to have a *tubal occlusion* immediately after you give birth, a local anesthetic is recommended because it is much less disruptive to breastfeeding than general anesthesia. A local anesthetic is preferred at this time because general anesthesia and any heavy sedation are associated with reduced milk production for as long as 2 weeks. Anesthetic drugs show up in the breast milk and appear to interfere with the establishment of a good sucking response, which can cause problems with breastfeeding.

If this permanent form of contraception has been carefully considered beforehand, immediately after childbirth is a good time to have the procedure, because the uterus and fallopian tubes are high in the abdomen and are easier for the surgeon to reach. This means the incision can be very small, the tubes need little manipulation, and the uterus does not have to be pushed up with an instrument.

Vasectomy is always an excellent method if no more children are wanted, because of its effectiveness and lower cost. However, counseling is especially important if a couple is making this decision shortly before or after the birth of a child.

Although progestin-only methods—Depo-Provera, progestin-only pills, and Norplant—are safe, they are not the methods of first choice for breastfeeding women, because the hormones do show up in breastmilk. No negative effects, however, have been documented so far among children exposed to these hormones as breastfed infants. Progestins do not negatively affect milk production or an infant's growth and health.

Nevertheless, starting a progestin-only method while nursing should be delayed until at least 6 weeks after the birth, for these reasons: (1) There is no risk of ovulating during these weeks. (2) This delay avoids exposing the newborn to hormones at the time when the baby theoretically might be more sensitive to them.

Combined oral contraceptives are not recommended if you are breastfeeding. The estrogen in the combined pill decreases the milk supply which usually leads to an earlier use of supplemental feeding and an early end to nursing. You can use progestin-only pills for the first 6 months and then switch to the combined pill, which is more forgiving if you do not use it perfectly.

Fertility awareness methods often are not recommended after childbirth and during nursing. Basal body temperature patterns generally are erratic and cannot be used to predict ovulation. Cervical mucus patterns also may vary during this period and changes in mucus are much harder to detect. However, a recent study demonstrated that the symptothermal method can be used successfully—by women who were experienced in using it—to identify most of their fertile days (which were verified by hormone measurements). However, abstinence was necessary 25 to 50 percent of the time. It should be noted that these women were not new users of this method, and they were supported by their partners and by trained fertility awareness counselors.

In general, barrier methods are the best complements to nursing, because they have no impact on the infant and their reliability is enhanced by the contraceptive effect of breastfeeding.

18

Abortion

A woman is fertile for about 30 years of her life. If she has a normal reproductive system, becomes sexually active in her teens, and uses no contraception, she could have more than a dozen children. As a result, for most of her reproductive years the average woman is trying either to postpone or to avoid pregnancy.

More than half the 6 million pregnancies that occur in the United States each year are not intended. Of these mistimed or unwanted pregnancies, about 1.5 million are ended by an induced abortion. By the time they reach menopause, two-thirds of American women have had at least one unintended pregnancy, and many have had an abortion. Women who have abortions come from all religious, socioeconomic, and ethnic backgrounds.

According to researchers at the Alan Guttmacher Institute, 47 percent of all unwanted pregnancies happen to couples who practice birth control. The very small percentage (10 percent) of men and women who do not use contraceptives account for the remaining 53 percent of unintended pregnancies.

Almost all induced abortions in the United States take place between the 7th and 13th weeks of pregnancy (counting from the first day of the last menstrual period), which is in the first trimester

(3 months) of a pregnancy. Surgical abortions are not usually performed before the 6th week because the embryo is too small to find easily. The safest time to have a surgical abortion is before the 8th week. A first trimester medical abortion, a new technology using drugs instead of surgery, is usually performed before the end of the 8th week (before the 56th day of pregnancy).

The surgical method used most frequently for first trimester abortions is *vacuum aspiration*, also called *suction curettage*. Current medical alternatives use either *mifepristone* (formerly known as RU486) or *methotrexate*. Both are combined with *misoprostol*, a prostaglandin.

After the 13th week, a pregnancy is in its second trimester and the method used to end a pregnancy at this stage is *dilation and evacuation*. As each week of pregnancy passes, the risk of complications from an abortion increases and so does the cost. Abortions after 20 weeks usually are performed only if the fetus has a severe malformation or when it is necessary to save the life or health of the mother (Figure 18.1).

Although some abortions are performed in hospitals, most are carried out in clinics as outpatient procedures. The majority of clinics limit their services to the early months of pregnancy. (Only

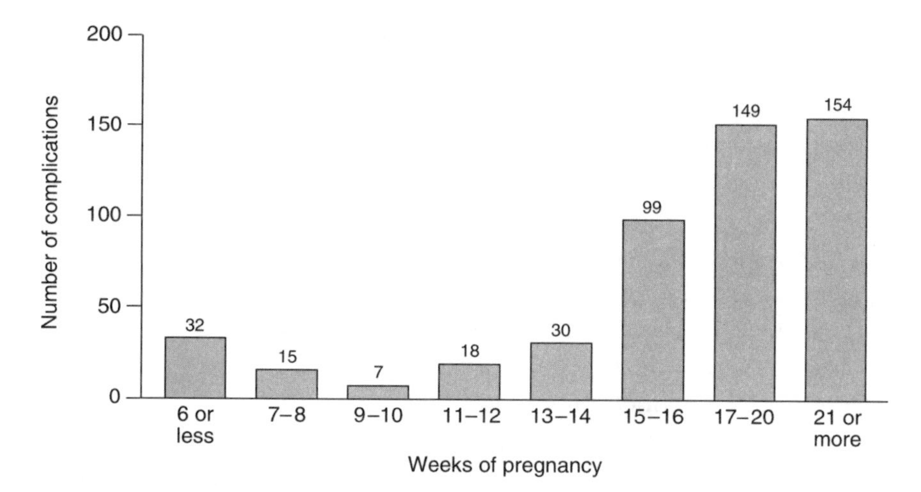

FIGURE 18.1 Serious Complications for Every 10,000 Abortions
Source: Stewart, Guest, et al. (1987).

IN A NUTSHELL

ABORTION

Today, both surgical and medical abortions are available. Surgical abortions most often use a suction technique to empty the uterus. Medical abortions use pills to make the uterus empty itself.

Surgical abortions take less time and at this time are still easier to obtain. Medical abortions are only available for very early pregnancy. They cause cramps and you will observe more bleeding. Both types are safe.

If you are considering an abortion, it is important not to delay. The earlier it is done, the easier it is and there is less chance of complications. Later abortions take longer and may require a hospital stay.

If you need help in getting a pregnancy test or finding a clinic that performs abortions, call the National Abortion Federation hotline: 800-772-9100.

25 percent of abortion providers perform such surgery after the 16th week of pregnancy.)

In the late 1980s, the office of the Surgeon General, having reviewed more than 250 studies, found no support for claims that legal abortion causes women emotional damage. They did note, however, that a woman's distress is greatest *before* an abortion and that most women reported feeling relieved and calm afterward, especially following a first trimester abortion.

Legal abortions are safe: the mortality rate for surgical abortions has remained at less than 1 death per 100,000 abortion procedures through the 1980s, according to the U.S. Centers for Disease Control.

HAVING AN ABORTION

You should start looking for an abortion provider right away if you think you may need an abortion. In large cities, this usually is not difficult, but in many states there may be only one source—or none at all. The quickest way to find help may be the National Abortion Federation hotline: 800-772-9100.

The First Step: A Pregnancy Test

You can find out if you are pregnant by testing yourself at home with a kit that can be bought at most drugstores. These tests are reliable if you follow the directions carefully. If the test is negative but you still do not have your period, you need a professional test. In fact, a good first step is to go to a clinic or a doctor for a pregnancy test and to do this as soon as you suspect you are pregnant. It is inexpensive, and the people you talk to are not likely to be judgmental.

The early laboratory test for determining pregnancy—a blood test—is so sensitive it can detect the very low levels of the pregnancy hormone, human chorionic gonadotropin, in your blood as early as 7, 8, or 9 days after fertilization. (The old standard urine test cannot confirm a pregnancy until 28 days after ovulation, when a menstrual period is about two weeks overdue.)

In addition to the blood test results, a pelvic examination is

PREGNANCY TESTS AND ABORTION: PROTECTING YOUR PRIVACY

If you are considered legally underage in your state (which usually means 18 years or younger), and you want to talk to a clinic about an abortion or having a pregnancy test, and are worried about privacy, here are some questions to ask. Some of these questions also are useful if you want a contraceptive method that requires the services of a clinic or doctor (the Pill, Norplant, Depo-Provera, a diaphragm, or cervical cap).

- Do you take care of people who are under 18 years old?
- Do my parents or another adult have to come with me?
- Do I need my parents' or another adult's permission to have (a pregnancy test), (an abortion), (this method of birth control)?
- Who will get the results of my pregnancy test? When will the results be ready?
- Will a bill for a pregnancy test be sent in the mail to my home? Can I pay for it in cash?
- If I want an abortion and the law says my parents or another adult must be informed, will you help me talk to them or find an alternative through the court system?
- Do you have someone who can answer my questions?
- Can I come back more than once to talk to someone about having an abortion? (Get as much counseling as you need.)

A NOTE OF CAUTION

Antiabortion groups may advertise in the Yellow Pages and elsewhere as family planning centers or even abortion providers or counselors. Their staff will try to discourage you from terminating your pregnancy and may deliberately delay you until it is late to obtain an abortion. Make certain the clinic you contact actually performs abortions before you make an appointment.

necessary to confirm the results and to estimate how far along the pregnancy is. Whether you are considering an abortion or will continue with your pregnancy, an accurate dating of the pregnancy is important. If your physician cannot determine how far advanced the gestation is, an ultrasound evaluation may be necessary. As early as 6 weeks after your last normal period, ultrasound can reveal a pregnancy sac inside your uterus, making it possible to know how long you have been pregnant.

Even with the early test, the window of time available for making a decision about a pregnancy is small. Most women realize they are pregnant at about six weeks. Because abortion is easier, safer, and much less expensive when done in the first trimester, this does not allow much time for assessing your feelings about having a baby, about your partner, and about your life situation.

The best place to get a pregnancy test is from a physician or clinic that can also provide you with objective counseling and help you carry out whatever decision you make about continuing the pregnancy. Good family planning clinics and doctors offer information on abortion, or where to go for prenatal care and, if you wish, adoption procedures. If the test shows that you are *not* pregnant, this type of clinic or health care provider can help you find a dependable method of birth control. *Wherever you go for a pregnancy test, make sure it is understood that you need an immediate appointment to verify a pregnancy.* If you will have to wait more than a few days for an appointment, find another doctor or clinic.

Because it is so important not to put off getting a pregnancy test, if you do not have ready access to a clinic that provides a range of family planning services, obtain a pregnancy test from your family doctor or your gynecologist. Although you own doctor may not perform abortions, a pregnancy test is a routine lab procedure. If you ask, the doctor may also help you find a reputable provider of family planning services that include abortion.

If you do not have a doctor and there is no Planned Parenthood clinic, the county health department or a nearby hospital may offer pregnancy testing, abortions, or information on clinics that provide abortions. In some cities, there may be an independent laboratory that offers pregnancy testing.

Finding a Clinic or Physician

Freestanding clinics are the most common providers of abortion services. Because many abortions are performed in these facilities, the attending physicians are extremely skilled in the procedures. One of their rules is that you must make your own decision about your pregnancy without any outside pressure. They believe they chiefly should offer objective and nonjudgmental information and counseling about your available options.

Not every community has a facility that offers abortion services. To find sources of abortion care elsewhere, start with your family doctor or gynecologist. Even if your doctor is uncomfortable doing abortions, he or she may (or may not) be willing to refer you to a surgeon or clinic that offers counseling and abortion care.

At colleges and universities, nursing personnel at the infirmary or the health service may be knowledgeable about pregnancy testing and what options are available. Just how much assistance they can provide, however, varies from school to school.

Planned Parenthood clinics are the most reliable sources of reproductive health services that include abortion. They will be listed in the white pages of the telephone directory. If there isn't one in your community, state or county health departments, departments of social services, or the Visiting Nurse Association traditionally provide the names of family planning clinics or medical practices that include abortion among their health care services. The departments of obstetrics and gynecology at most nondenominational hos-

THE NATIONAL ABORTION FEDERATION HOTLINE

An important resource is the National Abortion Federation (NAF), which operates a nationwide abortion hotline. By calling **800-772-9100** (toll-free), you can get answers to questions about abortion regulations in your state, the names of the nearest clinics that provide abortion services, including medical abortions, and suggestions on where to obtain financial help. (In Washington, D.C., the NAF number for abortion information is a local number, 202-667-5881.) The NAF will give out only the names of its affiliated clinics, which maintain high standards for care and counseling.

pitals may know of the nearest clinics that offer skilled abortion services. You can also try the Yellow Pages under "Clinics," "Abortion," or "Family Planning Information Centers." Finding help may not be easy, but it can be done if you are persistent and resourceful.

If There Are No Clinics in Your Area

The majority of U.S. counties do not have a facility that offers surgical abortions. If clinics or doctors in your area do not provide abortion services, call telephone information for the number of the Planned Parenthood affiliate in the nearest large city. Planned Parenthood clinics offer a broad range of family planning services, including abortion referrals. All their clinics must meet the organization's high standards for care and counseling, and some offer abortions.

Do not delay your search for good-quality abortion services, but do not act in a panic, either. If it appears that you will have to travel to another community or even to another state to obtain care, be certain that you are pregnant before you make your arrangements. Knowing how far the pregnancy has advanced gives you some idea of what procedures you will need—not all clinics offer second trimester procedures, for example—and this information will help you choose an appropriate clinic.

Although abortion is legal in the United States, each state has laws that regulate it. These laws may require a waiting period, an informed consent procedure, or the consent of parents if you are a minor. Many states restrict the availability of abortion or where it can be done when pregnancies have advanced beyond certain weeks. The National Abortion Federation hotline is the best source of information about restrictions in your state.

How to Check Out a Clinic

As with any other facility that offers health care, a clinic or surgeon providing abortion services should meet certain standards. Ask questions when you visit the clinic or doctor for the first time. Questions to ask include:

- Do they have a *written* agreement with a nearby hospital to provide backup emergency care if necessary? How many minutes away by car or ambulance is the hospital? (It should be within a 10 to 20 minute drive, preferably closer.) Do clinic physicians have admitting privileges at that hospital? Does the clinic have the capability of transferring a patient to the hospital?
- Are private spaces set aside in the clinic for talking with clients? Is printed information available on fees and on the availability of public assistance or other funds? Does the information on fees itemize the services included in the basic fee, and does it list the additional services that might be needed and their costs?
- Is the recovery room supervised at all times by either a licensed nurse or a physician who is on the premises?
- Does the facility have on hand a "crash cart"—the utility cart that holds the equipment for providing cardiac and pulmonary resuscitation? Is at least one staff person on each shift trained in cardiopulmonary resuscitation (CPR)?
- Are drugs on hand to treat cardiac arrest, an asthma attack, an allergic reaction, a seizure, or shock?
- Is the operating room large enough to hold several people as well as the equipment? Is it well-lighted? (Ask to see it.)
- Is there an adequate supply of intravenous solutions and at least six units of plasma volume expander available for emergency use? (The expander is used as a blood substitute to maintain blood pressure in case of hemorrhage.)
- Is there a sterilizing facility for the instruments?

• Does the clinic routinely send aborted tissue to a pathology laboratory to confirm that pregnancy tissue was indeed removed, if it cannot be identified visually? (A positive result means the pregnancy was in the uterus and is not an ectopic pregnancy still growing in a fallopian tube or some other place outside the uterus, where it could rupture.)

• If this is a second trimester abortion, is diagnostic ultrasound available? An examination by ultrasound is recommended before *any* second trimester pregnancy is terminated. After the 14th week, the National Abortion Federation requires that its member clinics perform an ultrasound examination for an exact determination of fetal size and position. Some states also may require this of abortion facilities.

With the availability of vacuum aspiration (suction) equipment, there is no need today for surgeons to perform first trimester abortions with a sharp curette, and few do. Because some physicians may still use this method, however, it is a worthwhile precaution to ask the doctor what method he or she uses. With a suction curette, pain and bleeding are reduced and the risk of leaving pregnancy tissue behind is decreased. Some clinics now offer a medical abortion, which uses drugs instead of surgery, as well.

What Happens at the Clinic

Although the procedure before an abortion varies from clinic to clinic or surgeon to surgeon, in general it should cover the same points. A medical assistant or counselor will answer your questions and work with you to determine whether you need more information or other help in deciding what to do. She or he will want to make certain that you have considered all your options and are comfortable with your decision. If the clinic offers medical abortions, this method will be described so you can make an informed choice about which approach you may prefer. Together you will go over the lengthy informed consent document you must sign before the abortion can take place. The counselor should be able to answer all your questions about the clinic's emergency preparations and facilities, about the procedures, and what happens afterward. *As most counselors will tell you, at any point before the abortion actually gets under way, you can change your mind.*

The counselor or medical assistant will take your medical history. You will be asked about any allergies to local anesthetics, antibiotics, common pain relievers, and other drugs. You also will be asked about current illnesses or conditions that might affect the performance of the abortion.

If you have decided to have an abortion, an appointment will be made for the procedure, and several tests will be performed, including:

- A blood or urine pregnancy test.
- A blood count to check for anemia.
- A blood test to determine if you are Rh negative. If you are, you will be given Rh immune globulin after the abortion to avoid the risk of Rh sensitization, which could have an adverse effect on a later pregnancy. (This procedure is done for every pregnancy, whether carried to full term or not.)
- Clinic rules may require that you be tested for gonorrhea, syphilis, chlamydia, or the AIDS virus. If you have an active STD, the clinic is likely to treat the disease before scheduling your abortion, so that the abortion procedure does not spread it to the upper part of your reproductive system. In addition, some clinics test for sickle cell disease and cancers of the reproductive tract.

If you are having a surgical abortion and are allergic to the lidocaine family of local anesthetics, general anesthesia may be advised. General anesthesia might also be preferable if you have any problem that makes it difficult for you to be calm and cooperative when surgery is performed with a local anesthetic. If you have any medical condition that might increase the risk of complications during the procedure, the clinic may suggest that a hospital is a better place for having the abortion. Such a condition might be a bleeding disorder, severe asthma, heart disease, severe diabetes, or epilepsy that is not well controlled.

Before a Surgical Abortion

At most clinics you will receive instructions about what to do to prepare for the abortion. You will be given pregnancy and blood tests, and a brief physical. If the clinic uses osmotic dilators to help open the cervix, these are inserted the day before the procedure. Osmotic dilators are short, slender, and made of a highly absorbent material. As they absorb moisture, they gradually expand, gently enlarging the cervical opening. They are put in while you lie in the usual position for a pelvic exam. Because some cramping can occur during the insertion, a local anesthetic may be injected. Without such anesthetic some women have no discomfort, while others experience mild cramps. In the rare event that you have severe pain or bleeding after the dilators are in place, call the clinic or the doctor who will be doing the abortion.

You will be given instructions about how long to avoid food and drink before the surgery, depending on the type of anesthesia that will be used.

Take a shower or bath just before you leave for the clinic. Arrange to have a friend or relative who knows about your pregnancy go with you to provide emotional support and to take you home. You will be at the facility for several hours and much of that time may be spent waiting, so you may also want to bring something to read or to do. After the abortion, if your friend cannot drive you home, plan to take a taxi.

At the clinic, the physician who is going to perform the procedure will conduct a brief examination, which includes checking the size and position of the uterus to determine again the size and length of the pregnancy. As we have said, if your pregnancy is over 14 weeks, many clinics do an ultrasound check to confirm the size of the fetus. Some clinics perform ultrasound whenever the pregnancy is thought to be over 12 weeks.

THE SURGICAL PROCEDURES

The abortion technique used will depend on the length of the pregnancy. In the first 3 months, a suction or "vacuum" method is used; a pregnancy between 3 and 6 months requires a dilation and evacuation procedure; later abortions are rare and are special cases that require special treatment.

First Trimester Vacuum Aspiration

The first trimester of a pregnancy is the first 3 months—12 to 13 weeks—counting from the first day of your last menstrual period. The most commonly used method of abortion during this period is the vacuum aspiration method, also called vacuum curettage or suction curettage. (Curettage means "scraping out," aspiration is "removal by suction.") Vacuum aspiration is similar to the method used by dentists to remove saliva and blood from your mouth. It safely and effectively empties the uterus through the opening in the cervix.

Although occasionally there are medical or psychological reasons to use general anesthesia, a vacuum aspiration most often is carried out with a local anesthetic. It can be performed in various outpatient settings: clinics, private medical offices, surgicenters, or hospital outpatient centers.

The cervix must be dilated to approximately one-half inch in diameter in order to insert the vacuum tube (cannula). For an early abortion, the tube is about the diameter of a drinking straw. The opening in the cervix can be enlarged with a metal dilator at the time of the surgery or by using an osmotic dilator beforehand, as described above.

At the time of the abortion itself, a speculum is placed in the vagina and the cervix is disinfected. A speculum is made of metal and looks like a bit like a duck's bill. It is designed to spread and hold open the vagina so the cervix can be seen. It seldom causes pain, although it is not very comfortable. Pain-carrying nerves are made numb next with injections of lidocaine or a similar anesthetic. Because the cervix has widely spaced nerve receptors, you may not feel the injection at all, although it sometimes can set off cramps that usually pass quickly.

After the anesthetic has taken effect, the physician gently grasps the cervix with an instrument called a tenaculum and, if necessary, dilates it further until it is open enough to accept the suction tube. The duration of the pregnancy determines the size of the tube—more advanced pregnancies require a larger tube. The tube is connected by a hose to an electric vacuum pump, like those used by dentists. If the pregnancy is less than nine weeks, some clinics simply use a large syringe for suctioning.

During the aspiration, the tube is moved around inside the uterus to loosen and remove the pregnancy sac and the thickened lining of the uterus. This takes a few minutes; more advanced pregnancies will require more time. The tube is removed, and the inside of the uterus is gently explored with a curette, a loop-shaped instrument with sharp edges, to make sure all the tissue has been removed. The suctioning takes 3-5 minutes and the entire process requires 10 to 15 minutes.

Discomfort or pain caused by the vacuum procedure varies. Some women feel almost nothing; others find it quite uncomfortable. Toward the end, when most of the tissue has been removed, the uterus contracts. This causes cramps that can range from mild to severe. Fortunately, they seldom last for more than an hour and can be relieved by medication. Most women feel well enough to walk out of the procedure room. Besides cramping, it is not unusual to have some vaginal bleeding and nausea afterward; nevertheless, most women feel ready to go home within an hour or so.

After the Surgery

If you have had an outpatient procedure, you should not be discharged until you have recovered satisfactorily. While you are still in the recovery room, the attending nurse or doctor should check your pulse, blood pressure, how much vaginal bleeding you are having, and your general physical condition. If a general anesthesia was used, you should be fully alert before you are discharged. Before you leave, make an appointment for a followup examination. Also get an emergency telephone number in case a complication develops after the clinic or office closes.

You may feel like returning to your usual level of activity immediately, or you may want to take it easy. Generally speaking, it is a

DANGER SIGNS AFTER SURGICAL ABORTION

Immediately contact your surgeon or the clinic where you received your abortion, or go to the nearest hospital emergency room, if you experience these symptoms:

- a temperature over 100.4 degrees Fahrenheit;
- chills, fatigue, or overall aching feeling;
- cramps or abdominal pain that steadily worsens;
- an abdomen that feels tender or painful when touched or when you cough, sneeze, walk, or jump;
- bleeding that lasts more than 3 weeks, or bleeding that for 3 days is more than your usual, heaviest, menstrual flow;
- unusual or bad-smelling vaginal discharge; or
- pregnancy signs that do not disappear.

good idea to avoid strenuous exercise for at least a few days. Showering immediately after the abortion is all right, but do not take a bath for several days to avoid the risk of introducing bacteria into the uterus.

Expect some cramps and vaginal bleeding during the next weeks. It is normal for light bleeding or spotting or just brownish discharge to occur off and on for as long as a month afterward. If the bleeding is heavy—if you are soaking more than one sanitary pad an hour and/or passing clots larger than a half dollar—and it lasts for more than 1 or 2 days, call the clinic or physician who performed the abortion.

The cramps that usually follow an abortion almost always respond to over-the-counter pain relievers. A non-aspirin product is a better choice because it does not interfere with blood clotting. The standard dose of two tablets every 3 or 4 hours usually provides relief. If your cramps are so severe that this does not help, or if the pain becomes steadily worse, call your clinic or doctor.

The drug methergine may be prescribed during the first 24 to 48 hours after the abortion to encourage firm uterine contractions and limit the amount of bleeding. If this results in severe cramps or pain that spreads downward to your thighs, call your practitioner. To ease the cramps it may be necessary to stop taking the drug.

Because infection is possible after a surgical abortion, take your temperature if you have chills or feel feverish. If you are taking a pain reliever such as acetaminophen, take your temperature *before* you take the pills, because they lower body temperature. If you have a temperature over 100.4 degrees F, call your physician or the clinic.

Do not use tampons (use sanitary pads), douche, or have intercourse for 2 weeks after the abortion to avoid the possibility of infection. If you have had a late (second trimester) abortion, you may develop breast milk. To stop it, wear a snug-fitting bra day and night for 2 or 3 days. Avoid any stimulation of the nipples and do not squeeze the milk from your breasts, since this increases milk production.

Second Trimester Dilation and Evacuation

The second trimester is the second three-month period of a pregnancy—between 14 and 26 weeks of gestation. Ending a pregnancy after 14 or 15 weeks is more complicated because the fetus is larger and there is a greater blood supply to the uterus. Only about 10 percent of abortions in the U.S. are carried out in the second trimester, and most are done during the first few weeks of this period.

The procedure most commonly used at this stage of a pregnancy is called dilatation and evacuation, or D&E. The cervix must be dilated to a greater degree—to more than half an inch—because the fetus is larger. Dilating the cervix may take more time, and the abortion itself takes longer. This technique is preferred for pregnancies that are between 13 and 16 weeks, and very skilled surgeons may use it for pregnancies that are up to 20 weeks or even longer. It is safer than an instillation abortion, which can also be used for second trimester pregnancies. Like vacuum aspiration, a D&E can be performed in outpatient settings, as long as there is hospital backup readily available. If it is carried out later in this trimester, it is often done in a hospital.

Having a D&E is much like having a vacuum aspiration, although with an increased risk of complications. If local anesthesia is used, the amount of discomfort and the sensations are very similar, and the recovery time is about the same. If general anesthesia is used, there is no pain or discomfort, but the recovery time generally is longer.

In these later abortions, osmotic dilators generally are used to open the cervical canal. At the time of the procedure, after the anesthetic has taken effect, such dilators are removed and, if necessary, the cervical canal is expanded further with a surgical dilator.

In a D&E, a larger vacuum tube is necessary. It is used in combination with a forceps and other instruments that break up pieces of tissue and remove anything that cannot be suctioned out. To minimize blood loss, surgeons may use drugs to encourage the uterus to tighten up or contract. A dilation and evacuation takes 20 to 30 minutes. It is the safest method for ending a second trimester pregnancy and is used for the majority of these advanced pregnancies.

Seldom-Used Surgical Methods

Instillation Abortion. A long, hollow needle is inserted through the abdominal wall and into the liquid-filled amniotic sac surrounding the fetus. A solution of salt or prostaglandin hormones is slowly instilled through the needle into the pregnancy (amniotic) sac. These can be combined or used alone to induce labor so the fetus and placenta are expelled. Until the 1970s, instillation abortion was the most common method for terminating second trimester pregnancies. Today it has been largely replaced by the safer and much shorter D&E.

An instillation abortion is almost always done in a hospital and can require 1 or 2 days of hospitalization. Osmotic dilators are sometimes inserted beforehand to help open the cervix. After the instillation, there is usually a wait of several hours or more before labor starts. Labor can be long and painful and generous amounts of pain medication may be needed.

After the fetus and placenta are expelled, pain and discomfort usually subside. If the placenta is not expelled completely, a D&C (dilatation and curettage) may be necessary. After an hour or two of rest, many women feel well enough to shower. Most hospitals require that women who have this procedure remain at least 3 to 4 hours afterwards for observation.

Hysterotomy. Hysterotomy is a major operation, somewhat like a mini-cesarean section, that requires general or epidural anesthesia. (Epidural is an injection into the epidural area of the middle/lower back.) A hysterotomy has a higher complication rate (and thus a higher death rate) than other methods. Moreover, any future pregnancies carried to term may require a cesarean delivery, because a hysterotomy incision is thought to weaken the uterus wall. (Unlike a true cesarean section, the incision is made in the upper part of the uterus, where it is more likely to rupture during another labor.) Hysterotomies were used for second trimester abortions during the brief period right after abortions were made legal everywhere in the United States and before other methods became readily available. Today they are limited to the extremely rare second trimester cases in which a woman has a uterus so seriously malformed that a D&E would be dangerous.

Hysterectomy. Hysterectomy, the removal of the uterus itself, also is a major surgery that requires an epidural or general anesthesia. It, too, carries a substantial risk of complications and a higher mortality risk. Today a hysterectomy is considered inappropriate for abortion and should be performed only when no other procedure is possible.

Menstrual Extraction. Not strictly an abortion method, in menstrual extraction a syringe was used to remove the contents of the uterus when a woman feared she was pregnant, such as after a missed menstrual period or rape, without waiting for a urine test to confirm this. Menstrual extraction was used before the availability of the blood test that can detect a pregnancy as early as 8 days after conception. With the development of this test and the increasing availability of emergency contraception, menstrual extraction is no longer needed.

COMPLICATIONS FROM SURGICAL ABORTIONS

Before 1973, when abortion became legal in the United States many women died or had serious medical problems after attempting to induce their own abortions or by going to untrained practitioners who performed abortions with primitive instruments or in unsanitary conditions. Women ended up in emergency rooms with serious complications: perforations of the uterus, retained placentas, severe bleeding, cervical wounds, rampant infections, shock, and gangrene.

Today, serious complications from abortions done during the first trimester are unusual. Of the 3 percent of women who have complications, 2.5 percent have minor complications that can be handled in the physician's office or at the clinic. Approximately 0.5 percent require an additional surgical procedure and/or hospitalization.

Complication rates are somewhat higher for abortions performed between 13 and 24 weeks. General anesthesia, if it is used, also carries a risk. In addition to the length of the pregnancy, important factors that affect the possibility of complications include the skill and training of the practitioner, the kind of anesthesia used, the woman's health, and the method used.

Hemorrhage. The most common complication immediately after an abortion is excessive bleeding. Of every 1,000 women who have abortions, between 2 and 10 have profuse bleeding. A very small percentage bleed so severely they need a transfusion. Excessive bleeding occurs when the uterus is not completely cleared of pregnancy tissue or when it does not tighten up enough afterwards. Bleeding also can occur if the uterus, cervix, or vagina have been injured. Heavy bleeding usually is prevented by using a drug to encourage the uterus to contract (its contraction closes the blood vessels) and by using a local rather than a general anesthetic. General anesthesia appears to reduce the strength of uterine contractions and is associated with greater blood loss. Making sure all the placenta has been expelled or removed from the uterus also helps prevent blood loss. It is especially important that this be done thoroughly in a second trimester abortion, when the uterus is bigger and tissue is more apt to be overlooked.

Substantial blood loss also can occur if a blood vessel has been cut or damaged accidentally during the procedure. If the blood loss is not great and the tear (in the cervix, for example) can be repaired with stitches, the abortion can be completed. If the injury is severe, it is best dealt with in a hospital. A transfusion may be necessary and exploratory surgery or laparoscopy may be needed to determine the extent of the damage.

In fewer than 1 percent of cases, blood clots can accumulate in the uterus, requiring another suctioning procedure. If you have a bleeding disorder or are taking medication that may slow blood clotting, you are at greater risk of hemorrhage.

Incomplete Abortion. An abortion is not complete if any tissue remains in the uterus. Most obvious indications of an unfinished abortion are cramps and bleeding. If you continue to experience signs of pregnancy—nausea, breast tenderness, and fatigue—seek treatment.

In some instances of incomplete abortion, however, you may have no signs of pregnancy or any other indications that the abortion was not thoroughly done. For this reason, it is important to see your surgeon for your post-abortion examination, which generally is scheduled when you have your abortion. If it will be difficult to return to the clinic where you had the abortion, arrange to have this checkup performed by a local doctor or other health care provider.

Infection. Cramps, pain that gets worse, fever, a smelly vaginal discharge, pelvic discomfort, and feeling unwell may be signs of an infection in the uterus or fallopian tubes. The presence of tissue fragments in the uterus increases the risk of infection.

If you suspect an infection, seek medical care at once. Most infections respond well to antibiotics if they are caught early. An infection that becomes severe can require hospitalization and vigorous treatment with intravenous antibiotics. Infections of the uterus and fallopian tubes may cause scar tissue and adhesions to form, making it difficult or impossible to become pregnant in the future. Severe infections can necessitate a hysterectomy and the loss of the uterus, fallopian tubes, and ovaries.

To avoid this risk, many clinics routinely provide an antibiotic just before or for 1 or 2 days after the abortion. Women at risk for pelvic inflammatory disease may be given antibiotics longer. In addition, antibiotics are often prescribed beforehand for women with a heart valve disorder, an artificial heart valve, or another congenital heart abnormality. If you have one of these problems, discuss the use of antibiotics with the surgeon performing the abortion and, if possible, your heart specialist.

Injuries to the Uterus, Cervix, or Nearby Organs. In rare instances (fewer than 1 percent), the cervix is torn during the abortion and may require stitches. Such injuries are less likely to occur when laminaria are used to dilate the cervix. The wall of the uterus (or other organs) can be injured by an instrument. Simple puncture wounds are likely to close up and heal themselves, but if the instrument goes through the wall and damages other structures, emergency surgery may be required.

Drug Reactions and Other Adverse Effects. A reaction can be caused by the Novocain-like local anesthetics that may be used, by antibiotics, or by the drugs used for encouraging contractions.

In an instillation abortion, the saline solution can be injected accidentally into a blood vessel, causing death. Also, a blood vessel or the uterus can be injured by the needle. If saline mistakenly is injected into muscle, it may destroy the tissue in the immediate area.

Long-Term Complications. Abortions using suction, which are carried out early in the first trimester, appear to have no negative effects on a woman's future reproductive health. Such vacuum aspiration abortions do not increase the chance of having a miscarriage (spontaneous abortion), a premature birth, or a low-birth-weight baby in the future. Fertility also is not affected by an abortion that is carefully performed, especially when it is done soon after conception.

Complications after an abortion, however, especially an infection, can lead to infertility. Injuries to the cervix that occur during an abortion (or childbirth) can increase the chance of developing cervical problems during a future pregnancy. Such an injury may cause the cervical canal to weaken and open under the pressure of the growing fetus, causing a spontaneous abortion. Generally, this can be treated successfully.

MEDICAL METHODS

A medical abortion has the advantage of avoiding the complications that can arise from surgery and anesthesia. Although many women feel more comfortable with it, it requires one more clinic visit and the process takes longer than a surgical procedure.

The National Abortion Federation hotline (800-772-9100) can provide you with information on the nearest clinic or physician offering medical abortions.

Mifepristone (formerly known as RU486) with Misoprostol

The most commonly used drug combination for terminating early pregnancy worldwide is *mifepristone* plus *misoprostol.* Mifepristone blocks the action of progesterone and the maintenance of the implanted embryo. The embryo dies and is expelled by the uterus. This method works best during the early weeks of pregnancy. Later on, the placenta produces too much progesterone for mifepristone to counteract it effectively. Misoprostol is a prostaglandin that is a standard treatment for preventing gastric ulcers caused by the use of nonsteroidal anti-inflammatory medicines (such as aspirin and ibuprofen). It also causes the uterus to contract.

When used alone, mifepristone is 65 to 80 percent effective in terminating an early pregnancy. When it is combined with prostaglandin, the success rates for early first trimester abortions have exceeded 95 percent. Mifepristone combined with a prostaglandin has been used for abortions in France, Great Britain, China, Sweden, and other countries, and more than 350,000 women now have chosen this method.

In the United States, clinical trials involving more than 2,100 women in 17 medical centers have been completed. As of this writing, the data from these studies are being prepared for publication in a medical journal, and a New Drug Application (NDA) has been filed with the Food and Drug Administration. This method is not expected to be generally available until at least 1998.

In some countries this abortion method is used up to the 49th day, in others it is used to the 63rd day. Initially, in the United States, the FDA registration of the drug limited it to use up to the 49th day. Additional information may permit an extension to the 63rd day.

Mifepristone is given in three tablets, taken at the clinic. The woman returns 2 days later for two pills containing a dose of misoprostol. After taking the misoprostol, she must rest in the clinic for a few hours, during which time most women abort. If this does not occur in about 4 hours, she goes home and waits for it to happen sometime during the next 2 weeks. About three-quarters of the abortions take place during the first 24 hours after taking the misoprostol.

Vacuum aspiration may be required in the approximately 5 percent of cases in which the placental tissue is not completely expelled or, occasionally, because of excessive bleeding or because an abortion does not occur at all.

Most of the side effects of this treatment occur right after the misoprostol is taken. The effects of a single dose of misoprostol are cramps, abdominal pain, and bleeding like that of a heavy period. Some patients experience nausea, vomiting, and diarrhea that may be severe enough to require medication. Heavy bleeding may continue for a week; bleeding that is not heavy can last for 1 to 3 weeks. In rare cases of severe bleeding, a woman may require a surgical abortion and/or a blood transfusion. In Europe, 2 to 3 women out of every 1,000 who used this method have needed a transfusion.

In its 10 years of use in Europe, there have been few serious medical problems with this method of medical abortion. Because a small, single dose is used and most of it is eliminated from the body in a few days, the risk of long-term health effects is slim. Almost all healthy women who are not allergic to these drugs can have a medical abortion.

Mifepristone, when it becomes available, will not be sold over the counter or through a prescription. It will be distributed only to qualified physicians who have been trained in using this method and will be given to patients under direct medical supervision. This policy is designed to ensure that the physicians who provide these methods have the information they need to counsel patients, and also have the necessary backup medical services.

Methotrexate and Misoprostol

Very recently several clinical studies in the United States have shown that another drug combination can induce abortions successfully and safely during early pregnancy. In the studies, a combination of methotrexate and misoprostol was 90 to 95 percent successful when the pregnancy was 49 days or less, but the abortion took longer to complete than with the combination of mifepristone and misoprostol.

Methotrexate prevents cells from dividing and growing. It has been used safely for many years to treat unruptured ectopic pregnancies, some cancers, and some nonmalignant diseases such as psoriasis and rheumatoid arthritis. In the doses used for abortion, it is safe for most healthy women who are not allergic to it.

In this two-step method, after receiving either an injection or tablets of methotrexate, the woman is given a vaginal suppository of misoprostol to be used at home 5 or 6 days later. Many physicians suggest that the woman insert the suppository when she will be able to rest for some time, such as before bedtime or at the start of a weekend, because she can expect about 12 hours of hard cramping and brisk bleeding. Acetaminophen with codeine is prescribed for easing the cramps.

Fifty to 60 percent of women who have used this method had an abortion within 24 hours after inserting the misoprostol. Another 10 to 20 percent abort after using a second suppository. Those for whom the misoprostol is not effective immediately may have to wait 2 to 3 weeks before cramps begin, followed by bleeding.

If the drug regimen is unsuccessful, vacuum aspiration is used to empty the uterus. Only a very small percentage of women require this additional step.

Most women using methotrexate plus misoprostol bleed for 7 to

10 days afterward and have some spotting for an additional 3 to 5 days. About 5 weeks pass before they have a menstrual period, which is similar to the after effects of a surgical abortion.

This method currently is available only at medical centers where it is being studied.

Prostaglandins Used Alone

Prostaglandins are chemicals made naturally by the body that act much like hormones. Some have been copied in synthetic versions and have a variety of medical applications. Several stimulate the uterus to contract during labor, for example, and have been used alone as vaginal suppositories or as injections to terminate more advanced pregnancies—those that are between 12 and 24 weeks. Nevertheless, today a prostaglandin alone is rarely used—perhaps in 1 percent of cases. Usually second trimester pregnancies can be ended more easily and with fewer side effects by a D&E. But if a physician is not thoroughly experienced in the D&E technique, prostaglandin suppositories are a safer alternative because they do not require special surgical expertise. However, a D&C or a D&E still must be done if the prostaglandin fails to work, which happens occasionally. So a physician who does not perform these procedures must be prepared to transfer his patient to a surgeon who does.

If a suppository is used, it is placed high in the vagina, and the hormone is absorbed by the blood supply in the vaginal walls. These prostaglandins stimulate intense, painful contractions of the uterus. Compared to injections, suppositories have the advantage of being removable if a severe adverse reaction develops, before they are totally absorbed.

For advanced pregnancies, the dose of prostaglandin in each tablet needs to be high, and a new tablet usually must be inserted every few hours. The constant high dose frequently produces such side effects as extreme nausea, vomiting, and diarrhea. Such reactions often can be alleviated by medicine prescribed by the physician. About one-half of women who have abortions this way also exhibit a marked rise in temperature. An abortion by prostaglandin suppositories takes an average of 14 hours after the insertion of the first tablet.

A prostaglandin also can be administered as an injection or by an intravenous drip to induce labor contractions. This approach has many side effects and is not always effective. Like the suppository, it causes a high rate of vomiting and diarrhea. Ten to 20 percent of the women who receive prostaglandins alone in any form require a D&C afterward to remove placental tissue that was not expelled.

Contraception After Abortion

You need to start using a contraceptive method before you have sex again if you want to be sure you do not get pregnant. Most likely, your surgeon or the clinic counselor will bring up the subject; if they do not, raise the question yourself. If your pregnancy was the result of a contraceptive failure, you may want to change methods.

It is possible to be sterilized when you have an abortion if it takes place before the end of the 10th week of pregnancy, before the uterus becomes large and soft. However, it is only in large urban centers that you may find a clinic able to provide abortion and sterilization services simultaneously. Often, surgeons who perform sterilizations prefer to use general anesthesia, which requires hospitalization and is more expensive. For information on sterilization and vasectomy, see Chapters 12 and 13, and discuss this option with your physician or the counselor at the clinic.

COST

An early surgical abortion (before 10 weeks), using local anesthesia and performed in a clinic that does many abortions every year, costs an average of $300. Otherwise, costs can range from $140 (for subsidized care) to $1,700 or more, depending on where and when the abortion is done. The price increases sharply for second trimester abortions. Clinics will charge about $600 for an abortion performed at 16 weeks and $1,100 at 20 weeks. These fees can go as high as $2,500 at 16 weeks to $3,000 at 20 weeks, depending on where the procedure is performed. Hospital charges generally are at least several times higher than the fees charged by clinics that specialize in women's reproductive care. In addition, the use of general anesthesia sustantially increases the cost.

A medical abortion in a clinic will cost about the same as an early surgical procedure (about $300), largely because of the extra number of clinic visits that are necessary.

Except in New York, California, and Washington, D.C., Medicaid generally does not pay for abortions. Some health insurance plans cover the cost of abortions for employees and their dependents. Others pay only for abortions that are necessary for medical reasons. Health maintenance organizations (HMOs), in general, are likely to include abortions in their coverage. Whether your health insurance coverage includes this procedure depends on the individual company writing the insurance or on your particular plan. Many health insurance plans include abortion under maternity benefits.

If you do not know what your health plan coverage includes, get a copy of your benefits sheet from your company's personnel office or from the insurance company. (It may be easier to retain your privacy by talking to the insurance company.) You will need to know your benefits identification number or the name of your health benefits package (such as "Master Medical") when requesting information.

Employees of the U.S. government, including those in the armed services, are not covered for abortion services. Similarly, women who work for state or city governments also may not be covered for abortion by their health insurance.

If you do not have health coverage and cannot afford to pay for an abortion, there may be funds available to you in your community. Women's health groups or feminist groups may make loans or outright grants of money. The hotline of the National Abortion Federation (800-772-9100) has information on sources of financial assistance. In addition, state or local chapters of the National Abortion Rights Action League (NARAL) and the National Organization for Women (NOW) may have a fund earmarked for women who need abortion services. These chapters usually are listed in the white pages of your local telephone directory; if you cannot find them, call their Washington headquarters. (Not all states have chapters of these organizations.) The number of NARAL in Washington is 202-973-3000; for NOW it is 202-331-0066. Your local Planned Parenthood affiliate also may have access to private funding sources.

Counselors at abortion clinics also may be knowledgeable about the resources available in their community. Some cities may have little-known, private foundations that help women pay for abortions. If you need financial help, pursue the available resources early and vigorously.

Sources

Adler, N.E., H.P. David, et al. "Psychological Responses After Abortion," *Science* 248 (April 6, 1990):41-44.

Alvarez, F., V. Brache, et al. "New Insights on the Mode of Action of Intrauterine Contraceptive Devices in Women," *Fertility and Sterility* 49, no. 5 (May 1988):768-773.

American Medical Association. *Encyclopedia of Medicine.* New York: Random House, 1989.

Andrews, W.C. and K.P. Jones. "Therapeutic Uses of Oral Contraceptives," *Dialogues in Contraception* 3, no. 3 (Winter 1991): 1-8. Published by the University of Southern California School of Medicine, Los Angeles.

Antarsh, L. "AVSC Embarks upon a Program to Teach Local Anesthesia for Female Sterilization," *AVSC News* 27, no. 3 (October 1989):1-2. Published by the Association for Voluntary Surgical Contraception.

Beresford, T. *Unsure About Your Pregnancy?* Washington, D.C.: National Abortion Federation, 1990.

Billings, E. and A. Westmore. *The Billings Method.* New York: Random House, 1980.

Boston Women's Health Book Collective. *The New Our Bodies, Ourselves.* New York: Simon and Schuster, 1984.

Bracken, M.B. "Oral Contraception and Congenital Malformations in Offspring: A Review and Meta-analysis of the Prospective Studies," *Obstetrics & Gynecology* 76, no. 3 (September 1990):552-557.

Bracken, M.B., K.G. Hellenbrand, and T.R. Holford. "Contraception Delay After Oral Contraceptive Use: The Effect of Estrogen Dose," *Fertility and Sterility* 53, no. 1 (January 1990):21-27.

"Breastfeeding and Contraception," *Outlook* 8, no.1 (March 1990):2-10.

"British Study Suggests Long-Term Pill Use Before First Term Pregnancy Raises Risk of Breast Cancer," *Family Planning Perspectives* 19, no. 6 (November/December 1987.):267-269.

Broome, M. and K. Fotherby. "Clinical Experience with the Progestogen-Only Pill," *Contraception* 42, no. 5 (November 1990):489-495.

Brown, H.P. "The Pill and Breast Cancer," *Health and Sexuality* 1, no. 1 (Fall 1990):6-7.

"Can You Rely on Condoms?" *Consumer Reports,* March 1989, pp.135-141.

Cancer and Steroid Hormone Study of the Centers for Disease Control and the National Institute of Child Health and Human Development. "Oral-Contraceptive Use and the Risk of Breast Cancer," *New England Journal of Medicine* 315 (August 14, 1986) :405-411.

Cates, W., Jr., and K.M. Stone. "Family Planning, Sexually Transmitted Diseases and Contraceptive Choice: A Literature Update—Part I," *Family Planning Perspectives* 24, no. 2 (March/April 1992):75-84.

Cates, W., Jr., and K.M. Stone. "Family Planning, Sexually Transmitted Diseases and Contraceptive Choice: A Literature Update—Part II," *Family Planning Perspectives* 24, no. 3 (May/June 1992):123-128.

Cates, W., Jr., A.E. Washington, et al. "The Pill, Chlamydia and PID," *Family Planning Perspectives* 17, no. 4 (July/August 1985):175-176.

Centers for Disease Control and Prevention (CDC), National Center for HIV, STD, and TB Prevention, Division of HIV/AIDS Prevention. HIV/AIDS Surveillance Report 8, no. 2. (December 1996) Atlanta: Centers for Disease Control.

"Clients at STD Risk Need Barrier Methods," *Network*, Family Health International 14, no. 4 (May 1994):11-17.

Collaborative Group on Hormonal Factors in Breast Cancer. "Breast Cancer and Hormonal Contraceptives: Collaborative Reanalysis of Individual Data on 53,297 Women with Breast Cancer and 100,239 Women without Breast Cancer from 54 Epidemiological Studies," *The Lancet* 347 (June 22, 1996):1713-1727.

"Controversy Over HIV Protection Persists, Despite Promising Studies of Nonoxynol-9," *Contraceptive Technology Update* 15, no. 2 (February 1994):13-16.

Creinin, M.D. and M. Park. "Acceptability of Medical Abortion with Methotrexate and Misoprostol," *Contraception* 52 (1995):41-44.

Creinin, M.D and E. Vittinghoff. "Methotrexate and Misoprostol vs Misoprostol Alone for Early Abortion: A Randomized Controlled Trial," *Journal of the American Medical Association* 272 (1994):1190-1195.

Darney, P.D. "Hormonal Implants: Contraception for a New Century," *American Journal of Obstetrics and Gynecology* 170 (May 1994):1536-1543.

Darney, P.D., E. Atkinson, et al. "Acceptance and Perceptions of Norplant Among Users in San Francisco, USA," *Studies in Family Planning* 21, no. 3 (May/June 1990):152-160.

"Depo-medroxyprogesterone Acetate (DMPA) and Cancer: Memorandum from a WHO Meeting," *Bulletin of the World Health Organization* 64, no. 3 (1986):375-382.

"Diagnostic and Therapeutic Technology Assessment of Intrauterine Devices," ed. H.M. Cole. *Journal of the American Medical Association* 261, no. 14 (April 14, 1989):2127-2130.

"Do Studies Point to Real Breast Cancer Risk with OCs?" *Contraceptive Technology Update* 11, no. 5 (May 1990):69-70.

"Does Oral Contraceptive Use Lead to Delayed Contraception?" *Contraceptive Technology Update* 11, no.4 (April 1990):63-64.

Emergency Contraception Hotline. Booklet published by Reproductive Health Technologies Project, Washington, D.C.

"Family Planners: Beware of 'Lunatic Fringe Sperm,'" *Contraceptive Technology Update* 16, no. 6 (June 1995):71.

Farr, G., H. Gabelnick, et al. "Contraceptive Efficacy and Acceptability of the Female Condom," *American Journal of Public Health* 84, no. 12 (December 1994):1960-1964.

Fertility Control, ed. S.L. Corson, R.J. Derman, and L.B. Tyrer. Boston: Little, Brown, 1985.

"Findings of the 1996 CREST Study: AVSC Technical Statement." New York: AVSC (Association for Voluntary Surgical Contraception) International, April 1996.

Fotherby, K. "The Progestogen-Only Pill," in *Contraception—Science and Practice,* ed. M. Filshie and J. Guillebaud. London: Butterworths, 1989.

"FPA Announces New Advice for Progestogen-only Pill Users," United Kingdom Family Planning Association, July 5, 1996.

"A Fresh Look at Barrier Contraceptives," *Contemporary OB/GYN,* March 1988:132-152.

Gallagher, D.M. and G.A. Richwald. *Fitting the Cervical Cap: A Handbook for Clinicians*. Los Gatos, Calif.: Cervical Cap, Ltd., 1989.

"General Anesthesia for Female Sterilization Under Scrutiny," *Contraceptive Technology Update* 11, no. 2 (February 1990):28-30.

Gold, R.B. *Abortion and Women's Health: A Turning Point for America?* New York: Alan Guttmacher Institute, 1990.

Goldstein, M. "Vasectomy and Vasectomy Reversal," in *Current Therapy in Endocrinology and Metabolism—3*. Philadelphia: B.C. Decker, 1988.

Goldstein M. and M. Feldbert. *The Vasectomy Book*. Boston: Houghton Mifflin, 1982.

Grady, W.R. and K. Tanfer. "Condom Breakage and Slippage Among Men in the United States," *Family Planning Perspectives* 26, no. 3 (May/June 1994):107-111.

Graedon, J. and T. Graedon. *The People's Pharmacy*. New York: St. Martin's Press, 1996.

Grimes, D.A. "Intrauterine Devices and Pelvic Inflammatory Disease: Recent Developments," *Contraception* 36, no. 1 (July 1987):97-109.

Grimes, D.A. "IUD Insertion: A Clinical Refresher," *The Female Patient* 14, no. 2(1989):51-54.

Guidelines for Breastfeeding in Family Planning and Child Survival Programs, ed. M.H. Labbok, P. Koniz-Booher, et al. Washington D.C.: Georgetown University Press, 1990.

Guillebaud, J. *The Pill.* Oxford, England: Oxford University Press, 1980.

Guillebaud, J. "Advising Women Which Pill To Take," *British Medical Journal* 311 (October 28, 1995):196-197.

Guillebaud, J. "Tri-cycling, Bi-cycling, Late Starts and Missed Pills: Creative Ways to Manage OC Problems," presented at Contraceptive Technology Conference on Issues and Options in Reproductive Health Care, Washington, D.C., March 14-16, 1996.

Harlap, S., K. Kost, and J.D. Forrest. *Preventing Pregnancy, Protecting Health: A New Look at Birth Control Choices in the United States.* New York: Alan Guttmacher Institute, 1991.

Hatcher, R.A., J. Trussell, F. Stewart, et al. *Contraceptive Technology, 16th Revised Edition.* New York: Irvington, 1994.

Having an Abortion? Your Guide to Good Care. Washington, D.C.: National Abortion Federation, 1990.

Hausnecht, R.U. "Methotrexate and Misoprostol To Terminate Early Pregnancy," *New England Journal of Medicine* 333, no. 9 (August 31, 1995):537-540.

"The Health Benefits of Oral Contraceptives." *Contraception Report* 1, no. 3(1990):3-5.

Henshaw, S. "Factors Hindering Access to Abortion Services." *Family Planning Perspectives* 27, no. 2 (March/April 1995):54-59, 87.

Henshaw, S. and J. Van Vort. "Abortion Services in the United States, 1987 and 1988," *Family Planning Perspectives* 22, no. 3 (May/June 1990):102-143.

Hilts, P.J. "U.S. Is Decades Behind Europe in Contraceptives, Experts Report," *New York Times*, February 15, 1990.

"How Reliable Are Condoms?" *Consumer Reports*, May 1995:320-325.

Institute of Medicine. *Contraceptive Research and Development: Looking to the Future.* Washington, D.C.: National Academy Press, 1996.

"Is It Safe to Prescribe Oral Contraceptives Until Menopause?" *Contraceptive Technology Update* 10, no. 12 (December 1989):167-171.

Kaeser, L. "Reconsidering the Age Limits on Pill Use," *Family Planning Perspectives* 21, no. 6 (November/December 1989):273-274.

Kennedy, K.I., B.A. Gross, et al. "Breastfeeding and the Symptothermal Method," *Studies in Family Planning* 26, no. 2 (March/April 1995):107-115.

Klaus, Hanna. *Natural Family Planning: A Review.* Washington, D.C.: National Family Planning Center of Washington, D.C., Inc., 1995.

Koonin, L., K.D. Kochanek, et al. "Abortion Surveillance, United States, 1988," *Morbidity and Mortality Weekly Report* 40, no. SS-2 (July 1991):15-42.

"LAM 98% Effective, If Certain Rules Are Followed," *Contraceptive Technology Update* 17, no. 1 (January 1996):6.

"Latex Allergy Reaches Epidemic Proportions," *Contraceptive Technology Update* 16, no. 3 (March 1995):31-34.

Lee, N., G. Rubin, and R. Borucki. "The Intrauterine Device and Pelvic Inflammatory Disease Revisited: New Results from the Women's Health Study," *Obstetrics and Gynecology* 72, no. 1 (July 1988):1-6.

Li S., M. Goldstein, J. Zhu, and D. Huber. "The No-Scalpel Vasectomy," *Journal of Urology* 145 (February 1991):341-344.

McCann, M. and L. Potter. "Progestin-only Oral Contraception: A Comprehensive Review," *Contraception* 50, no. 6, suppl. 1 (December 1994):1-195.

McDonald, T.L. *The Cervical Cap Handbook.* Iowa City: Emma Goldman Clinic for Women, 1988.

Mills, A. "The Forgotten Progestogen Only Pill," *British Journal of Family Planning* 12 (1987):44-46.

"Minilaparotomy and Laparoscopy: Safe, Effective, and Widely Used." *Population Reports*, Series C, no. 9 (May 1985). Published by Johns Hopkins University.

"Minipills Remain Choice for 'Specialty Patient' Groups," *Contraceptive Technology Update* 9, no. 2 (February 1988):13-15.

Mosher, W.D. "Contraceptive Practice in the United States, 1982-1988," *Family Planning Perspectives* 22, no. 5 (September/October 1990):198-205.

National Research Council and the Institute of Medicine. *Developing New Contraceptives: Obstacles and Opportunities,* ed. L. Mastroianni, Jr., P.J. Donaldson, and T.T. Kane. Washington, D.C.: National Academy Press, 1990.

Natural Family Planning. Booklet by the Diocesan Development Program for Natural Family Planning, Washington, D.C.

"Natural Family Planning an Appealing Method for Some," *Contraceptive Technology Update* 11, no. 2 (February 1990):21-28.

Nelson, A.L. "Medical Complications and Birth Control: Diabetes, Cardiovascular Disease and Cancer," presented at Contraceptive Technology Conference on Issues and Options in Reproductive Health Care, Washington, D.C., March 14-16, 1996.

"New Label Broadens IUD Candidacy Profile," *Contraceptive Technology Update* 16, no. 5 (May 1995):59.

"New Studies Find No Link Between Spermicide Use and Heightened Risk of Congenital Malformations," *Family Planning Perspectives* 20, no. 1 (January/February 1988):42-43.

"No Increase in Risk of PID for IUD Users Who Are Married or Cohabiting with One Sexual Partner," *Family Planning Perspectives* 21, no. 1 (January/February 1989):35-36.

Norplant Contraceptive Subdermal Implants: Manual for Clinicians. New York: Population Council, 1990.

"Norplant: 'Most Effective Reversible Method in World'," *Contraceptive Technology Update* 11, no. 1 (January 1990):1-8.

Norplant Subdermal Levonorgestrel Implants: Guide to Effective Counseling. New York: The Population Council, 1992.

"The No-Sperm Vasectomy Failure," *Family Planning Perspectives* 26, no. 5 (September/October 1994):196.

"OC Compliance and Contraceptive Failure," *Contraception Report* 1, no. 4(1990): 3-6.

"On the Needless Hounding of a Safe Contraceptive," *The Economist*, September 2, 1995:75-76.

"Oral Contraceptive Association with Breast Cancer Is Not Conclusive, FDA Advisory Committeee Agrees; Recent Studies Do Not Support Labeling Change," *FDC Reports* 51, no. 2 (January 9, 1989):13-14.

"Oral Contraceptive Users May Be at Some Increased Risk of Cervical Carcinoma," *Family Planning Perspectives* 27, no. 3 (May/June 1995):134-136.

"Oral Contraceptives and Breast Cancer," *Health and Sexuality* 1, no. 1 (Fall 1990):1-5.

Ortiz, M.E. and H.B. Croxatto. "The Mode of Action of IUDs," *Contraception* 36, no. 1 (July 1987):37-53.

Overmyer, R.H. "In-Office Contraceptive Implant Is Effective, Long-Acting, Reversible," *Modern Medicine* 59 (January 1991):113-115, 119.

Pasquale, S.A. and J. Cadoff. *The Birth Control Book*. New York: Ballantine Books, 1996.

Petitti, D.B., S. Sidney, et al. "Strokes in Users of Low-Dose Oral Contraceptives," *New England Journal of Medicine* 335 (July 4, 1996):8-15.

Physicians' Desk Reference 50, Montvale, N.J.: Medical Economics Co., 1996.

"Pill Appears to Provide Long-Term Protection Against Endometrial Cancer and Ovarian Cancer," *Family Planning Perspectives* 19, no. 3 (May/June 1987):126-127.

"Pill Users Face Increased Risk of Cervical Cancer, But Decreased Risk of Other Genital Cancers," *Family Planning Perspectives* 21, no. 1 (January/February 1989):33.

Pollack, A.E. "Long-term Consequences of Female and Male Sterilization," *Contemporary Ob/Gyn* August 1993:45-46.

Pollner, F. "OC Age Limit Is Out of Date, FDA Advisory Panel Decides," *Medical World News*, November 27, 1989:12-13.

"Polyurethane Condom Could Attract New Users," *Contraceptive Technology Update* 16, no. 3 (March 1995):34, 39-40.

"Postcoital Contraception: A Necessary, Important Option," *Contraceptive Technology Update* 10, no. 11 (November 1989):145-153.

"Postcoital Contraceptives Available, But Seldom Used," *Contraceptive Technology Update* 10, no. 5 (May 1989):67-68.

Potts, M. "Birth Control Methods in the United States," *Family Planning Perspectives* 20, no. 6 (November/December 1988):288-297.

"Progestogens in the Pill Modify Levels of Serum Lipids, WHO Study Finds," *Family Planning Perspectives* 21, no. 3 (May/June 1989):141-142.

"Protective Effects of Oral Contraceptives Against Ovarian and Endometrial Cancers," *Contraception Report* 1, no. 3(1990):6-7.

Richwald, G.A., S. Greenland, et al. "Effectiveness of the Cavity-Rim Cervical Cap: Results of a Large Clinical Study," *Obstetrics and Gynecology* 74, no. 2 (August 1989): 143-148.

Rogow, D. and S. Horowitz. "Withdrawal: A Review of the Literature and an Agenda for Research," *Studies in Family Planning* 26, no. 3 (May/June 1995):140-153.

Schildkraut, J.M., B.S. Hulka, and W.E. Wilkinson. "Oral Contraceptives and Breast Cancer: A Case-Controlled Study with Hospital and Community Controls," *Obstetrics and Gynecology* 76, no. 3, pt. 1 (September, 1990):395-402.

Schlesselman, J.J. "Oral Contraceptives and Breast Cancer," *American Journal of Obstetrics and Gynecology* 163, no. 4, pt. 2 (October 1990):1379-87.

"Should Surgical Sterilization Be Considered Reversible?" *Contraceptive Technology Update* 10, no. 6 (June 1989):86, 88.

Silber, S.J. *How Not to Get Pregnant.* New York: Charles Scribner's Sons/Warner Books, 1987.

Silvestre, L., C. Dubois, et al. "Voluntary Interruption of Pregnancy with Mifepristone (RU 486) and a Prostaglandin Analogue," *New England Journal of Medicine* 322, no. 10 (March 8, 1990):645-648.

Sivin, I. "IUDs Are Contraceptives, Not Abortifacients: A Comment on Research and Belief," *Studies in Family Planning* 20, no. 6 (November/December 1989):355-359.

Soderstrom, R.F. *Male Sexual Health.* New York: Consumer Reports Books, 1991.

Stampfer, M.J., W.C. Willett, et al. "A Prospective Study of Past Use of Oral Contraceptive Agents and Risk of Cardiovascular Diseases," *New England Journal of Medicine* 319, no. 20 (November 17, 1988):1313-1317.

Standards for Abortion Care. Washington, D.C.: National Abortion Federation, 1988.

"Sterilization," *ACOG Technical Bulletin No. 222.* American College of Obstetrics and Gynecology, April 1996.

"Sterilization a Popular, Effective Method of Birth Control," *Contraceptive Technology Update* 11, no. 4 (April 1990):55-64.

Stewart, F.H., F.J. Guest, et al. *Understanding Your Body.* New York: Bantam, 1987.

Tatum, H.J. and S. Waldman. "The New ParaGard Copper T380A Intrauterine Device," *Medical Digest* 9, no. 1 (Winter 1989):1-5.

Thorogood, M. and M.P. Vessey. "An Epidemiologic Survey of Cardiovascular Disease in Women Taking Oral Contraceptives," *American Journal of Obstetrics and Gynecology* 163, no. 1, pt. 2 (July 1990):274-281.

Torres, A. and J.D. Forrest. "Why Do Women Have Abortions?" *Family Planning Perspectives* 20, no. 4 (July/August 1988):169-176.

Trussell, J. and K. Kost. "Contraceptive Failure in the United States: A Critical Review of the Literature," *Studies in Family Planning* 18, no. 5 (September/October 1987):237-283.

Trussell, J. and F. Stewart. "The Effectiveness of Postcoital Hormonal Contraception." *Family Planning Perspectives* 24, no. 6 (November/December 1992):262-264.

Trussell, J., R.A. Hatcher, et al. "Contraceptive Failure in the United States: An Update," *Studies In Family Planning* 21, no. 1 (January/February 1990):51-54.

Trussell, J., J.A. Leveque, J.D. Koenig, et al. "The Economic Value of Contraception: A Comparison of 15 Methods," *American Journal of Public Health* 85, no. 4 (April 1995):494-503.

Trussell, J., K. Sturgen, et al. "Comparative Contraceptive Efficacy of the Female Condom and Other Barrier Methods," *Family Planning Perspectives* 26, no. 2 (March/April 1994):66-72.

"The Truth About Abortion." Fact Sheet from the National Abortion Federation, Washington, D.C., 1996.

"U.S. Abortion Mortality," *Family Planning Perspectives* 25, no. 1 (January/February 1993):3.

U.S. Congress, Office of Technology Assessment. *Infertility: Medical and Social Choices.* Washington D.C.: U.S. Government Printing Office, 1988.

Utian, W. "Oral Contraceptives: Safe After 40?" *Patient Care*, March 30, 1989.

Van Look, P.F. "Postcoital Contraception," *Outlook* 8, no. 3 (September 1990):2-6.

Vessey, M.P., M. Lawless, et al. "Progestogen-Only Oral Contraception: Findings in a Large Prospective Study with Special Reference to Effectiveness," *British Journal of Family Planning 1985* 10:117-121.

Vessey, M.P., N.H. Wright, et al. "Fertility After Stopping Different Methods of Contraception," *British Medical Journal,* February 4, 1978.

Visness, C.M. and R. Rivera. "Progestin-Only Pill Use and Pill Switching During Breastfeeding," *Contraception* 51(1995):279-281.

Weil, M. and T.L. MacDonald. *Fertility Awareness: Natural Birth Control for Women.* Iowa City, Iowa: Emma Goldman Clinic for Women, 1982.

Weir, S.S., P.J. Feldblum, et al. "The Use of Nonoxynol-9 for Protection Against Cervical Gonorrhea," *American Journal of Public Health* 84, no. 6 (June 1994):910-914.

"Which Drugs Truly Interfere with the Efficacy of OCs?" *Contraceptive Technology Update* 10, no. 8 (August 1989):105-108.

"Which Patients May Benefit from Alternative Contraceptive Methods?" *Contraception Report* 1, no. 4(1990):7-12.

Whittemore, A.S., et al. "Characteristics Relating to Ovarian Cancer Risk: Collaborative Analysis of 12 U.S. Case-Control Studies: II. Invasive Ovarian Cancers in White Women," *American Journal of Epidemiology* 136 (1992):1184-1203.

WHO Collaborative Study of Cardiovascular Disease and Steroid Hormone Contraception. "Venous Thromboembolic Disease and Combined Oral Contraceptives: Results of International Multicentre Case-Control Study," *The Lancet* 346 (December 16, 1995):1575-1582.

WHO Special Programme of Research, Development and Research Training in Human Reproduction. "A Randomized, Double-Blind Study of Two Combined and Two Progestogen-Only Contraceptives," *Contraception* 25, no. 3 (March 1982):243-252.

"Who Will Provide Abortions?" Report of a national symposium sponsored by the National Abortion Federation and the American College of Obstetricians and Gynecologists. Washington, D.C.: National Abortion Federation, 1990.

Winikoff, B. "Breastfeeding," *Current Opinion in Obstetrics and Gynecology 1990* 2:548-555.

Winikoff, B., P. Semeraro, and M. Zimmerman. *Contraception During Breastfeeding.* New York: Population Council, 1989.

Wymelenberg, S. *Science and Babies: Private Decisions, Public Dilemmas.* Washington, D.C.: National Academy Press, 1990.

Index

L

M

N

S

T

BROOKLYN PUBLIC LIBRARY
3 4444 23087 7524